Handbook
of Remotivation Therapy

THE HAWORTH CLINICAL PRACTICE PRESS
The Haworth Handbook Series in Psychotherapy
Terry S. Trepper, PhD
Editor

Handbook of Remotivation Therapy edited by Jean A. Dyer and Michael L. Stotts

Handbook of Anger Management: Individual, Couple, Family, and Group Approaches by Ronald T. Potter-Efron

Titles of Related Interest:

Therapeutic Interventions for the Person with Dementia edited by Ellen D. Taira

The "Feeling Great!" Wellness Program for Older Adults by Jules C. Weiss

The Geriatric Patient: Common Problems and Approaches to Rehabilitation Management edited by Mary C. Singleton and Eleanor F. Branch

Rehabilitation Interventions for the Institutionalized Elderly edited by Ellen D. Taira

A Guide to Creative Group Programming in the Psychiatric Day Hospital by Lois E. Passi

The Clinical Treatment of the Criminal Offender in Outpatient Mental Health Settings: New and Emerging Perspectives edited by Sol Chaneles and Nathaniel J. Pallone

The Mentally Impaired Elderly: Strategies and Interventions to Maintain Function edited by Ellen D. Taira

Parkinson's Disease and Quality of Life edited by Lucian Côté, Lola L. Sprinzeles, Robin Elliott, and Austin H. Kutcher

A New Look at Community-Based Respite Programs: Utilization, Satisfaction, and Development edited by Rhonda J. V. Montgomery

Treating Co-Occurring Disorders: A Handbook for Mental Health and Substance Abuse Professionals by Edward L. Hendrickson, Marilyn S. Schmal, and Sharon C. Eckleberry

Addicted and Mentally Ill: Stories of Courage, Hope, and Empowerment by Carol Bucciarelli

Designing, Implementing, and Managing Co-Occurring Treatment Services for Individuals with Mental Health and Substance Use Disorders: Blueprints for Action by Edward L. Hendrickson

Jean A. Dyer, PhD
Michael L. Stotts, CAS
Editors

Handbook of Remotivation Therapy

Pre-publication
REVIEW

"**D**yer and Stotts have put together a handbook which highlights the development of a practice model in psychosocial counseling applied to a variety of health and mental health settings. Although today practice is more directly guided by outcome-driven analyses, this view of model development provides a process-driven analysis of interest to historical and conceptual development. This handbook gently reminds us that consumers often are less interested in the mechanics of psychotherapeutic interventions than in a clarity of ideas with the interventions that also communicate respect and hope."

Ronald J. Mancoske, DSW
Professor, School of Social Work,
Southern University at New Orleans

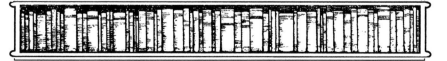

#32.50

Handbook
of Remotivation Therapy

Jean A. Dyer, PhD
Michael L. Stotts, CAS
Editors

250201

The Haworth Clinical Practice Press™
The Haworth Reference Press™
Imprints of The Haworth Press, Inc.
New York • London • Oxford

RC489.R43 H36 2005

0 1 3 4 1 0 7 6 3 5 2 1 8

Handbook of remotivation therapy /
c2005.

2005 04 27

For more information on this book or to order, visit
http://www.haworthpress.com/store/product.asp?sku=5191

or call 1-800-HAWORTH (800-429-6784) in the United States and Canada
or (607) 722-5857 outside the United States and Canada

or contact orders@HaworthPress.com

Published by

The Haworth Clinical Practice Press™ and The Haworth Reference Press™, imprints of The Haworth Press, Inc., 10 Alice Street, Binghamton, NY 13904-1580.

PUBLISHER'S NOTE
Identities and circumstances of individuals discussed in this book have been changed to protect confidentiality.

Cover design by Lora Wiggins.

Library of Congress Cataloging-in-Publication Data

Handbook of remotivation therapy / Jean A. Dyer, Michael L. Stotts, editors.
    p. ; cm.
    Includes bibliographical references and index.
    ISBN 0-7890-2470-5 (hard : alk. paper)—ISBN 0-7890-2471-3 (soft : alk. paper)
    1. Remotivation therapy—Handbooks, manuals, etc.
    [DNLM: 1. Mental Disorders—therapy. 2. Psychotherapy, Group—methods. 3. Motivation. WM 430 H2353 2005] I. Dyer, Jean. II. Stotts, Michael L.
RC489.R43H36 2005
616.89'14—dc22

2004012039

CONTENTS

ABOUT THE EDITORS

Jean A. Dyer, PhD, is Dean, School of Nursing and Health Sciences at Westminster College in Salt Lake City, Utah. Professor Dyer was associated with the National Remotivation Therapy Organization for five years. She delivered a formal presentation on the interdisciplinary application of remotivation therapy at the national organization's 2002 Annual Institute. Professor Dyer is the author of "Multidisciplinary, Interdisciplinary, and Transdisciplinary Teaching Models and Nursing Education," published in *Nursing Education Perspectives.* She also produced *Grief and the Older Adult: The Need to Care* through Health Sciences Consortium.

Michael L. Stotts, CAS, served as Executive Director of the National Remotivation Therapy Organization (NRTO) from 1994-2003. Prior to that position, he was an association executive in Washington, DC, a gerontological educator with several medical schools, and a research and advisory consultant to the U.S. Department of Health and Human Services. His career is marked by several years as an executive improving educational standards of health practitioners, principally long-term care administrators. In this role he created the first organized curriculum and degree program for administrators of nursing homes at the College of DuPage in Naperville, Illinois. He has organized over one hundred national meetings on subjects as diverse as centenarians and remotivation therapy, and international symposia on long-term care. At the present time, he is an educational consultant to several national membership organizations.

CONTRIBUTORS

John J. Allison has two degrees from LaSalle University and has training and experience in advanced group therapy. He is a United States Navy veteran and has held hospital chaplaincy positions in both acute care and mental hospitals. He has taught English at the secondary and collegiate levels. Now retired, he continues to work as a parish deacon.

John R. Bierma has worked as a case manager in mental health, an instructor in pre-retirement education, a behavioral consultant to long-term care facilities, a university professor, and as executive director of an area health education center. He currently serves as the director of a rural health network in northwest Mississippi. He has practiced and taught remotivation therapy for thirty years and has held various offices on the board of the National Remotivation Therapy Organization, Inc.

Cheryl Davis is a native of New York City currently working as a court-appointed guardian for adults in Raleigh, North Carolina. She is a graduate of William and Mary in sociology and has twenty years' experience working with adults and adolescents who have mental health, substance abuse, or physical health issues.

Nancy Farmer has twenty-two years' experience working with older adults, principally as a nationally certified activity professional. As a remotivation therapist, she is an instructor and has been a member of the board of directors of the Bay State Remotivation Council and the National Remotivation Therapy Organization. She has taught numerous activities and quality-of-life classes to health professionals.

Robert S. Garber is a psychiatrist and a past president of the American Psychiatric Association. Formerly, he was the medical director of the Carrier Clinic, a private psychiatric hospital in Bell Mead, New Jersey. He has also had many committee appointments in the American Psychiatric Association, including chair of the original committee that sponsored remotivation therapy.

Barbara Herlihy-Chevalier has nearly fifty years' experience in geriatric and psychiatric nursing. She has held many leadership positions in both the National Remotivation Therapy Organization, Inc., and the Bay State Remotivation Council, Inc., including president. For over three decades she has trained hundreds of health care professionals in basic and advanced remotivation therapy.

Jason J. Meixsell graduated from College Misericordia with honors and went on to become first vice president and then president of the National Remotivation Therapy Organization. Mr. Meixsell has completed the requirements for certification as a validation worker. He has taught remotivation therapy as an adjunct instructor at College Misericordia and has published articles on this topic.

James Siberski is the coordinator, Gerontology Education Center for Professional Development at College Misericordia and an adjunct instructor of psychiatry, School of Medicine, Pennsylvania State University. He has published various articles of interest to a broad range of health professionals including his concept of the psychosocial staircase. Since 1985 he has presented more than 100 workshops throughout the country on numerous topics including activities for the elderly, reminiscing therapy, suicide, elder abuse, Alzheimer's disease, remotivation therapy, and the psychosocial needs of the elderly.

Florinda R. Sullivan has developed, directed, and consulted in programs treating children and older adults. As a registered nurse, she has conducted several presentations both nationally and locally on topics as varied as the role of community health nurses as advocates, the needs of urban women, health and psychosocial needs of elders, the use of remotivation therapy with patients diagnosed with Huntington's Disease, and community-based nursing research. She is currently the clinical director of a home health agency in Tewksbury, Massachusetts.

Nancy Vandevender has been active in the field of geriatric recreation for twenty-three years. Her certifications include Certified Therapeutic Recreation Specialist (CTRS), Certified Remotivation Therapy Trainer, level II (CRmT II) from the National Remotivation Therapy Organization, Inc., and she is a certified instructor for NCCAP Basic and Advanced Management Courses. She has presented workshops on remotivation therapy, recreation programming, dementia care, self-defense, staff development, documentation, and exercise. She is a contributing editor to *Creative Forecasting*. Currently she is Director of Recreation/Volunteers at the Jewish Home of Greater Harrisburg, Pennsylvania.

Frances Kay Vickery is a psychologist with experience in the penal system and a state mental hospital. Dr. Vickery is also a statistician and a consultant in personnel testing and evaluation systems. She is certified in advanced group remotivation therapy and continues to do group work in retirement.

Foreword

The beginning of remotivation is well documented in this anthology, and the reader will find it rich in interesting detail. In the foreword I offer some of my thoughts and perceptions about its development and evaluation.

Smith Kline & French enjoyed the exclusive rights for marketing Thorazine in the 1950s and 1960s, and they generously supported the development of remotivation training programs and educational materials related to it nationwide. This became a large network of programs based particularly in state mental hospitals. Large numbers of regressed and withdrawn chronic mental patients benefited not only from the Thorazine they received but also from the positive resocialization achieved through the remotivation process. Many patients could live in open settings, or in less restrictive settings, at home, or in other community placement. We witnessed the onset of what came to be known as deinstitutionalization. Administrators of public mental hospitals could and did close wards that formerly housed chronic long-term psychotic patients. The hospitals themselves closed or became smaller, short-stay hospitals. An increasing array of psychotropic medications were used to quickly stabilize patients and return them to the community.

It might look as if remotivation therapists worked themselves out of jobs with the long-term chronic patient, but this was far from the end of the story. This anthology attests to the subsequent development of the National Remotivation Therapy Organization (NRTO) and its existence today as a meaningful resource in caring for people.

Soon after I joined the staff of the American Psychiatric Association (APA) in 1961, I became familiar with remotivation and the APA–Smith Kline & French (SKF) Remotivation Advisory Committee chaired by Dr. Robert Garber. Walter Pullinger from Philadelphia State Hospital led the national training center. I remember well the earnest and able leadership of Mr. Pullinger in the meetings of the advisory committee. At the time it was a happy and comfortable relationship that enjoyed the SKF functional support and the APA professional support of the wide network of remotivation trainers and therapists.

This relationship was not to last, however. SKF foresaw that its support would by necessity have to dwindle as its exclusive rights with Thorazine ended and many other competitive products came on the market. SKF sought to withdraw from supporting remotivation as gracefully as possible by asking the APA to take over with the help of a termination grant. Mr. Pullinger and a leadership group of remotivators were presented with the fact that the future of remotivation rested with their ability to become a viable independent organization. I pledged the support of the APA Mental Hospital Service (which later became the Hospital and Community Psychiatry Service) in planning for their independent organization, as well as revising and updating all education and training materials to provide an adequate supply of these for several years into the future.

In recent years psychiatry and the APA have moved away from their origins in public psychiatry toward a greater emphasis on private practice, oriented to what insurance benefits can provide for treatment. We know that the health insurance industry has resisted providing nondiscriminatory benefits for psychiatric patients. The time invested in caring for patients is often what helps them improve, yet this very "caring" is not considered a reimbursable treatment. In today's economic climate, progress is difficult. Too many priorities fight for available dollars. An endless imperative tells us to do more with less.

This present anthology about the history and practice of remotivation gives abundant testimony to the enduring benefits of this therapy in a wide range of hospital and community settings and its usefulness in treating a variety of conditions. It is not only a restorative modality that demonstrates how to recover intact areas of function that often lie hidden or dormant beneath overlying illness. It can also delay or prevent loss of function, as well as help maintain function that can easily slip away prematurely in the aging process for people with Alzheimer's, Huntington's, and similar chronic diseases.

There are still far too many nursing homes or other long-term care residential facilities or other living situations in which a pervasive insulation from meaningful life experience exists. A failure to maintain intact areas of functioning is the rule, not the exception. The principles of remotivation are part of the basic building blocks of caring for people in our society. I salute the NRTO leadership and its steadfast group of advocates for seeing that, notwithstanding past success, much more can still be done in bringing remotivation to those who can benefit from it.

I believe this anthology is a most useful documentation of past successes and of future challenges that lie ahead.

Donald W. Hammersley, MD
Deputy Medical Director (Retired)
American Psychiatric Association

Chapter 1

A Psychiatrist's View of Remotivation

Robert S. Garber

Why does remotivation work?

Ever since I became convinced that remotivation is good for patients, I've asked myself why. Here, in a tentative way, I'll try to answer that question. In looking for an answer, I needed to review a few fundamentals about mentally ill people, the ultimate purpose of those of us who work with the mentally ill, and the means we use to achieve that purpose.

In spite of the many diagnostic categories of mental illness, one single trait seems to characterize all mentally ill persons: they behave as though they live in a world different from the one in which the rest of us live. In their world, the absence of a smile may spell condemnation; a television set may be a brainwashing apparatus; a neighbor may be an agent of the devil. We are all familiar with highly elated patients who endeavor to cure the world's ills by writing checks for a billion dollars, depressed patients who believe that life is utterly hopeless, and patients who think that the FBI has recruited their spouses to spy on them.

From the moment that their concepts of reality change, mentally ill people do what is natural: they adjust to their new reality, just as we adjust to our reality. One patient uses an imaginary vast wealth for good causes. Another withdraws from a life that offers no joy or even hope. Other patients become secretive so that it will be harder for their families and the FBI to spy on them. In short, mentally ill people adjust to what they believe to be the facts of life.

Given this generalization, what is our ultimate purpose? By our purpose I mean the purpose of everyone on the psychiatric team—

Reprinted with permission from *Mental Hospitals*, American Psychiatric Association, Washington, DC, August 1965.

psychiatrist, nurse, aide—everyone who has contact with the mentally ill patient. To put it simply, we are trying to help mentally ill persons recognize the realities *we* recognize. We want them to see themselves for the persons they really are, to see other people as they really are, and to see relationships as they actually exist.

That is what we try to do, but we have learned that in dealing with the mentally ill we do not need to change patients completely in order to restore them to their families, jobs, and communities. In other words, we have learned that we do not need to cure them in order to send them home. Like the diabetic who must remain on insulin, the cardiac patient who needs digitalis, and the patient who loses a finger, the mentally ill person can become an ex-patient without being cured. When we send home a person who can function in the outside world, we have to a large degree achieved our purpose.

How have we done this? Basically, by establishing communication with the patients: by encouraging them to speak to us and by speaking to them. The underlying condition for this communication is, of course, trust. By one means or another we must inspire confidence, for without it we communicate the wrong message, and we reinforce the mentally ill person's distorted view of reality. We use this trust and communication to try to restore the patient's ability to recognize people, things, and relationships for what they really are. To help us do this we may use drugs, shock therapy, and other techniques—but every technique is directed at restoring reality to the patients.

We all communicate with patients, but we do not all do so in the same way. In fact, if we keep in mind that each patient is a many-sided human being, we might say that we communicate with different sides of the same patient. This requires us to use different techniques. My technique is psychotherapy. Yours is remotivation.

I said before that mentally ill patients have in common a distorted view of some significant aspects of reality. The key word here is *some*. Most mentally ill persons recognize, for example, that they are alive, so they will take nourishment as other living human beings do; many of them will complain appropriately if they get a toothache; many will dress appropriately for the weather, and so on.

We can say, then, that not every role they play is a sick role. It is sick when a patient puts a swastika on his forehead to keep his thoughts hidden from the psychiatrist, but there is nothing sick about his putting on boots to walk in the snow—if there is snow.

Each patient has sick roles and healthy roles. The sick ones have come to dominate his or her life, but the healthy roles are not entirely dead. I as a psychiatrist deal mainly with the sick roles. You as remotivators are in touch with the healthy roles. I deal with the patients' weaknesses. You deal with their strengths. These weaknesses and strengths are both contained in a single individual; they are as inseparable as the two sides of a coin. If we dealt only with weakness or only with strength, we would do little for the patient, because we ourselves would not have a clear, well-rounded view of reality: it would be distorted by our own one-sided approaches.

The patient's strength, as you know, can be very surprising, once you find it. You have considerable room for exploration, since every patient, like every other person, plays many roles: child, youth, brother, sister, student, parent, worker, housekeeper, reader, bowler, neighbor, club member, driver, eater, drinker, lover, traveler, thinker. The list is almost endless, and it grows as we age. Many of these roles may be distorted; others may become obscure; others may go on seemingly unaltered; and new ones may emerge. The totality of all these roles gives the patient—just as it gives all of us—a sense of identity, of uniqueness, of individuality.

These are the simple, fundamental thoughts I found useful to keep in mind in trying to discover why remotivation works. I believe that remotivation works because it recognizes mentally ill people as I have just described them.

Remotivation, from the very beginning, tells the patient that he or she is accepted as an individual, a man or woman with a name, with specific features, with many roles, with unique traits that distinguish him or her from everyone else. The patients who are recognized so specifically have already been reached, in a way. They have been told that among the hundreds or thousands of patients in this hospital, their faces and names are recognizable. They are not lost in the shuffle; they are not confused with someone else. In spite of the inevitable regimentation in almost every institution, they stand out; they are known to important people, that is, to the staff. The ability to do this for the patient is a reflection of the remotivator's own self-image, as Hildegard Peplau pointed out in her fine book, *Basic Principles of Patient Counseling.* Although she was writing of nurses, her concepts are applicable to everyone who comes in contact with patients. Peplau advocates for respect for the patient by treating him or her with the courtesy accorded a stranger. The nurse must be comfortable as a person and a professional in order to help patients accept their own independence and be constuctive problem solvers.

Why is this good for the patients? The changes in some of their old roles, and their new roles as mental patients, have altered their sense of identity and have created confusion for them. They may believe that their identities have been stolen from them or have suffered some kind of injury. Take the patient who is guilt ridden and depressed. He is sure that his sins make him an outcast. A remotivator says to him, "Nice to see you, Mr. Jones. Glad you've come." The remotivator shakes his hand. How does Mr. Jones interpret this? He may say to himself, *This man doesn't know how rotten I am. When he finds out . . .* However, the remotivator has plenty of time to find out, and he continues to treat Mr. Jones politely, warmly, cheerfully. The remotivator has brought him a new awareness. Not only the remotivator but other staff members treat him this way. There is some chance, then, that Mr. Jones will need to take another look at himself. He may be confronted with the possibility that he is not as bad as he thought, or that he was pretty bad but has reformed. One of the great values of remotivation is that it emphasizes to the patients that they have an objective existence to other people: not an existence that depends only on what the patients think of themselves, but one that depends to a large degree on how we, their fellow beings, see them.

If remotivation emphasized only the objective identity of the patient, it might not be really effective. Remotivation creates a bridge between the patients as they appear to the world and the patients as they appear to themselves. It does so by encouraging them to browse around in the concrete world and to identify and assert their experiences in interactions with other human beings. The only restriction you place on their browsing is that they must, in remotivation, come up with concrete, specific information. They must describe their experiences concretely. A patient must say, "This is how I built cabinets at the factory," or "It used to take me three days to plow one-hundred-fifty acres," or "Cactus plants need less water than other houseplants."

The patient must participate in this interaction as a plumber, a gardener, a sign painter, sailor, salesperson, geography teacher, cab driver, or in some other healthy role. The result is that the patients are strengthened in two ways. First, they are encouraged to describe themselves concretely and accurately as individuals with specific social functions, jobs, a place in the world. Second, they are encouraged to speak concretely and accurately of what they did in these jobs.

While the remotivator tries to build up the patient's sense of certainty in the concrete facts of his or her life, the psychiatrist tries, you might say, to reconstruct the patient's recognition and understanding of himself or herself and the world in which he or she lives. You can see how these two efforts complement each other.

That, in short, is why remotivation works—because it helps set in motion two processes that are vital to the patients if reality is to be restored to them. First, it builds on the patients' strengths, reinforcing them as objective people in our eyes and, in respect to their healthy roles, as subjective people in their own eyes. Second, remotivation works because the psychiatrist tries to challenge the distortions of reality that plague the patients. Put another way, remotivation works because it is a useful experience to the patients. They learn that there are roles they can play that do not create problems for them, that do not fill them with anxiety. They find that they do not need to block out or revise their understanding of every area of their lives, that some areas can be shared with a certain amount of freedom, competence, dignity, and even pleasure. In this way the texture of their lives does not get altogether lost. The smell, touch, and feeling of reality remain recognizable for them. They are not permitted simply to abandon themselves by abandoning, one by one, all the roles that made their lives meaningful; they are encouraged to keep them alive. This is what patients need, and this is why remotivation works.

We as mental hospital workers are obligated to be realists. Some patients were getting well before remotivation appeared on the scene. In fact, they were getting well long before psychiatry evolved. However, I would venture a good guess that they got well because their recognition of reality was somehow strengthened, and their distortions of reality were overcome. The corrective processes that were put in motion were like the ones we put in motion today. That is entirely understandable, since we human beings probably have not changed much in the few thousand years of history. We have, however, developed a better understanding of mental illness and, at the same time, a better understanding of how to treat it.

What the healers of ancient times relied on, I believe, was their intuitive sense of what the mentally ill person needed, combined with a natural sensitivity and artfulness in communication, and, of course, persistent optimism.

To this day, in my opinion, those same attributes characterize the best psychiatrists, psychiatric nurses, psychiatric aides, adjunctive therapists, and everyone else involved in understanding and communicating with the mentally ill. This, therefore, is the final reason for the workability of remotivation: *the remotivators.* You cannot separate technique from technicians. A fact of life is that a technique is no better than the man or woman who uses it, and it often turns out that the technician is really much better than the technique. In the last analysis, after all the techniques are outlined, the science behind them is verified, and the art of application is recognized, remotivation works because the remotivator—regardless of his or her title or condition of service—makes it work.

REFERENCE

Peplau, H.E. (1964). *Basic principles of patient counseling.* Philadelphia, PA: Smith Kline & French Laboratories.

Chapter 2

Remotivation:
The First Fifty Years

Jason J. Meixsell

Dorothy Hoskins Smith, an English teacher from Claremont College in California, developed remotivation therapy in the 1950s. The technique has evolved and today remotivation is a valuable therapy. This chapter provides a historical account of the inception of remotivation therapy and discusses the path that remotivation has taken over the past fifty years as well as what the future may hold.

DOROTHY HOSKINS SMITH

Dorothy Hoskins Smith moved from California to Massachusetts during World War II. She began volunteering at the Northampton, Massachusetts, Veterans Administration (VA) Hospital where she developed remotivation therapy to assist the people with whom she was working. As part of her volunteer work, Ms. Smith was asked to develop a public speaking course. She decided to use poetry as part of her approach. She probably chose the modality of poetry because of her background as an English teacher, but the reading of poetry had a tremendous impact on the residents. Most of the residents with whom Ms. Smith worked were catatonic and considered to be mute since they had not spoken in years. Ms. Smith read poetry and would ask the residents questions about the poem.

Bierma (1998) relates an account of Ms. Smith's first session with seven men in the VA hospital who hid under a grand piano when she began reading the poetry. Although most people would have considered this a failure, Ms. Smith sat next to the piano, instead, and continued to read the poem. The men slowly began to come out from under the piano and sit in on the group. Several members of this group answered the questions that she had asked about the poem and one had even asked for the poem to be read again. Ms. Smith believed that the strong rhythmical nature of the poems caught the attention of the group members and stimulated them. Another characteristic of poetry is that it worked with the physical and emotional aspects that were not affected by the residents' diseases. Working with the areas that were not affected by disease—called the unwounded areas by Ms. Smith—became an important tenet of remotivation therapy as it developed.

PHILADELPHIA STATE HOSPITAL

Based upon her success Ms. Smith decided to teach others the technique that she had developed. Many hospitals throughout the country declined training in remotivation saying that there was no credence to the technique and that the results that she had achieved were due to her positive personality. Dorothy Smith did not give up her quest and she continued to train in remotivation. A big break, however, came in the summer of 1956 when she was invited to give a presentation at Philadelphia State Hospital where a nurse, who worked with regressed residents, challenged Ms. Smith to get any of her people to respond. Ms. Smith conducted a remotivation therapy session with them, and according to an account given by McCormick (Bierma, 1998), several of the residents responded to her handshakes with smiles and assisted her by reading her poems. This account states that remotivation therapy training classes began at Philadelphia State Hospital the next day.

Remotivation therapy flourished at this hospital to such an extent that it became the national training center for remotivation. Ms. Smith trained many staff, most of whom were psychiatric aides at the hospital. It was thought, at that time, that remotivation therapy would best be conducted on the units by psychiatric aides because previously these workers had performed mostly custodial care, and remotivation could incorporate the aides into the therapeutic team as well as increase and strengthen the interaction between the residents and the aides (Robinson, 1967). Ms. Smith stayed at Philadelphia State Hospital for three months and trained approximately 200 psychiatric aides and other members of the treatment team in remotivation therapy (Cater et al., 1994). Later in 1956, a grant from the Mental Health Association of Southeastern Pennsylvania and from Smith Kline & French laboratories was used to expand the training using Philadelphia State Hospital as a national training center.

In February 1957, Smith Kline & French produced a training film on remotivation therapy that featured Smith. In the film, Ms. Smith discusses the five steps in a remotivation therapy session and demonstrates each step with a group of patients. Also included is a comparison between remotivation therapy and the other services that were offered at Philadelphia State Hospital. Remotivation therapy was used as a preparatory therapy with those who were not yet able to participate in higher forms of therapy such as psychotherapy. According to the film, psychiatric aides would evaluate the performance of those in the remotivation groups and consult with psychiatrists to discuss when a person was ready to be discharged from remotivation to a higher form of therapy (Meixsell, 1999).

According to Robinson (1967), Ms. Smith was scheduled to return to Philadelphia State Hospital in September 1957 to conduct additional remotivation therapy training classes. Unfortunately, Ms. Smith unexpectedly died earlier that year.

WALTER F. PULLINGER JR.

In October 1957, the completed film on remotivation was presented, along with a demonstration of remotivation therapy, at the Mental Hospital Institute in Cleveland, Ohio (Bierma, 1998). Although Ms. Smith's death did slow the plans for remotivation therapy, a new leader emerged. Among the original aides that were trained by Ms. Smith was Walter F. Pullinger Jr. Mr. Pullinger, who is also featured in the remotivation film conducting a session with residents, assumed the leadership role of remotivation therapy at Philadelphia State Hospital and continued Ms. Smith's teachings of remotivation.

Throughout the 1960s, Mr. Pullinger conducted remotivation therapy training classes at Philadelphia State Hospital, where he was named coordinator of remotivation in the United States and Canada. According to Bierma (1998), Mr. Pullinger was instrumental in the development of the original seventeen training centers for remotivation therapy.

In addition to his training in remotivation, Mr. Pullinger also worked to further develop the technique of remotivation therapy. He introduced variations of remotivation including sequential remotivation and wrote several articles about the technique and its success in mental health hospitals. He also wrote several books on remotivation sessions, and his book, *Poems for Remotivation,* is still utilized by remotivation therapists throughout the world. Because of his tremendous contributions to remotivation therapy, Walter F. Pullinger Jr. is affectionately recognized as the "father of remotivation."

TRAINING IN REMOTIVATION

In 1958, the Smith Kline & French Foundation created the remotivation project in order to conduct remotivation therapy training classes throughout the country. Also in 1958, an exhibit on remotivation therapy was shown at the American Psychiatric Association Annual Meeting (Cater et al., 1994). The Mental Hospital Service of the American Psychiatric Association developed an advisory committee for the remotivation project. This committee produced the first remotivation therapy training manual, written by Alice Robinson, then director of nursing at Vermont State Hospital. This manual outlined the history of remotivation to that point, provided the theory and process of remotivation therapy, and provided information on teaching and developing a remotivation program. This text, with the other materials listed, helped to spread remotivation throughout the United States and Canada.

In 1967, a textbook written by Allen Gibson and published by F. A. Davis Company provided further information on remotivation therapy. In the first chapter, the author stated that at the end of 1965 there were 241 remotivation programs in forty-five states and over 15,000 trained remotivators (Gibson, 1967). These numbers showed the growth of remotivation since Dorothy Hoskins Smith began teaching the technique in 1956.

NATIONAL ORGANIZATION

With remotivation therapy continuing to grow, a national organization for remotivation therapy was formed in 1971. This organization, the National Remotivation Therapy Organization (NRTO), provided the standards for remotivation therapy training and practice. In 1972, Walter

Pullinger was elected the first president of NRTO, and he was reelected in 1973. In the mid-1980s, the organization changed its name to the National Remotivation Therapy Organization to show that remotivation was not only a technique but a viable therapy. In 1989, NRTO became incorporated in the state of Massachusetts where the home office had been relocated. With the move of the national headquarters to Massachusetts, the national organization was now housed in the state where Dorothy Hoskins Smith had first used the therapeutic technique.

DECLINE OF REMOTIVATION

As stated earlier, remotivation therapy grew tremendously in the first ten years after its creation. Remotivation continued to flourish throughout the 1960s and hit its peak in the early 1970s.

A drastic decline in remotivation therapy occurred during the mid-1970s. This was due in large part to the deinstitutionalization movement, a nationwide effort to discharge people from state psychiatric facilities and to provide their care in settings that were based more in local communities. Many psychiatric hospitals were closed during the 1970s because patients were moved to community nursing homes.

Remotivation therapy training was drastically reduced. The technique of remotivation apparently did not move into the new community-based psychiatric treatment settings, which is evidenced by a drop in the number of active remotivators from the statistics given by Gibson (1967) to approximately 400 remotivators in the late 1990s (NRTO database, 1998). At this point remotivation therapy became confined to a few pockets of activity (Pennsylvania, Massachusetts, Tennessee, New York, North Carolina, and Wisconsin).

REMOTIVATION TODAY

Gibson (1967) referred to remotivation therapy as a therapeutic modality useful for health care providers in mental hospitals, as well as those working in other types of institutions. Although the idea was established that remotivation therapy could be used in other settings in addition to psychiatric facilities, remotivation training continued to be promoted in state mental health hospitals. This practice contributed to the near demise of remotivation therapy.

The 1980s and 1990s brought about an exploration of remotivation therapy in alternative settings. The most common sponsors of remotivation therapy training were in long-term care facilities for older adults. The result has been a focus on the psychosocial well-being and quality of life of older adults in long-term care facilities.

The principle of remotivation that states people can lead productive, fulfilling lives in any setting is being used to heighten the quality of life of those individuals who are fortunate to have this resource in their lives. All age groups are currently benefiting from participating in remotivation therapy sessions. Remotivation therapy is being used in conjunction with rehabilitation from physical illnesses or injuries in order to provide psychosocial support and intervention to increase the gains seen during rehabilitation. It is also being used with specific populations, such as those with Huntington's disease, Alzheimer's disease, and dementia; people with developmental delays due to mental retardation and substance abuse; as well as with other populations discussed in this text.

The technique of remotivation therapy is being used in special settings such as adult day care facilities, day treatment facilities, prison systems, senior centers, long-term care community nursing homes, rehabilitation facilities, child day care centers, and settings in the mental health system. The practitioners of remotivation therapy have been broadened to include not only nursing and psychiatric aides but also recreational therapists, activities directors, psychiatrists and psychologists, occupational therapists, social workers and case managers, clergy members, speech and language pathologists, and lay volunteers.

REFERENCES

Bierma, J. (1998). *Remotivation group therapy: Handbook for the basic course.* York Harbor, ME: National Remotivation Therapy Organization, Inc.

Cater, M., Lahaie, N., Lippert, E., and Sharkey, H. (1994). *Remotivation therapy: A group method that promotes rehabilitation.* Montreal, Quebec: The Association of Remotivation Therapists of Canada.

Gibson, A. (1967). *The remotivators' guide book.* Philadelphia, PA: F.A. Davis.

Meixsell, J. (1999). *Workbook of remotivation for the basic course.* York Harbor, ME: National Remotivation Therapy Organization, Inc.

NRTO database (1998). York Harbor, ME: National Remotivation Therapy Organization, Inc.

Robinson, A. (1967). *Remotivation technique.* Philadelphia, PA: Smith Kline & French.

Chapter 3

What Is Remotivation Therapy?

Barbara Herlihy-Chevalier

Remotivation therapy is objective in nature and is grounded in a philosophy that goes deeper than surface techniques. It is assumed that each person has a set of values which makes him or her important and worthwhile as an individual and member of society.

As defined by the National Remotivation Therapy Organization, Inc. (NRTO),

> Remotivation is a technique of simple group therapy, objective in nature, used with a group of patients in an effort to reach the "unwounded" areas of each patient's personality and to get them thinking about reality in relation to themselves. Remotivation differs from other therapies because it focuses on the patients' abilities rather than on their disabilities. The major endeavor is to discuss and develop the patient's healthy aspects no matter how regressed they may be. (Bierma, 1998, p. 9)

In the 1940s, Dorothy Hoskins Smith, a teacher of English literature, became a volunteer at a VA hospital in Northampton, Massachusetts. She worked with mute clients using poetry and rhythm. This process motivated these mute clients to respond and interact during sessions. Following her successes in Massachusetts, Smith was challenged to use her technique in a Pennsylvania psychiatric hospital with regressed clients. She was very successful and consequently established training programs designed with the psychiatric aide in mind.

Remotivation therapy allowed the psychiatric health care technician to be more than a custodian of patients. As a result, nonprofessional caregivers were able to use a therapeutic technique that helped to keep their patients alert and participative in their own care. In addition, lay volunteers have found remotivation therapy helpful because it provides a format through which they too can work constructively with various patients. Once certified in remotivation therapy, the volunteer can become an active, supportive member of the health care team.

Health care professionals and health administrators soon recognized remotivation therapy as a credible and cost-effective therapeutic modality. Nurses, activity directors, occupational therapists, and other discipline-specific health care providers became well versed in motivating their clients through the implementation of remotivation therapy techniques. Outcomes such as increased patient participation in planned activities of daily living, care planning sessions, and social interaction have made remotivation therapy an integral part of effective patient plans of care.

In some health care organizations, remotivation therapy requires a physician's order. Physicians well acquainted with the benefits of remotivation therapy can provide the needed support a reluctant client might require as he or she begins the remotivation process. Physicians, hospital staff, and nursing home administrators have come to realize that remotivation is a flexible technique that is cost effective and can be adapted to any facility's organizational structure. Remotivation therapy encourages an attitude of hope and enthusiasm on the part of all participating health care team members.

Every remotivation program must have a certified remotivation therapist, commonly called a "remotivator." The basic remotivation therapy course is designed to be competency based. To successfully complete the course and be certified as a basic remotivation therapist, one must attend a four-day basic course; demonstrate the methods to peers; develop complete remotivation sessions; conduct sessions with peers and volunteer patients; plan and implement twelve remotivation sessions as a practicum; and submit all twelve plans to the instructor for review and feedback (Bierma, 1998).

Remotivation therapy uses group discussion as its primary methodology. Its overall goals are to increase socialization and increase self-esteem. Each remotivation session features a group leader who introduces a specific topic and includes five distinct steps:

1. *The Climate of Acceptance* establishes a nonthreatening, warm, and friendly relationship in the group through touch, eye contact, and personal interaction.

2. *A Bridge to Reality* introduces a topic that would be relative to the group through the reading of objective poetry.
3. *Sharing the World We Live In* develops the topic through planned, open-ended, objective questions and presentation of sensory aids.
4. *An Appreciation of the Work of the World* is designed to stimulate the group members to think about work in relation to themselves as well as about work they may have done. It also covers the subjective aspects of the topic as people discuss past experiences, opinions, and values, and relate to the current environment.
5. *The Climate of Appreciation* provides a brief summary of the session, expresses pleasure in getting together, and invites group members to future meetings (Mental Hospital Services, 1956).

Remotivation sessions are usually held once a week, lasting from thirty minutes to an hour, depending on the attention span of the group members. On average six people are selected for each group, with criteria for reaching those who may be withdrawn, isolated, depressed, bored, or in need of environmental stimulation. It is multiscopic in that participants may be of low, average, or high functioning, and multidisciplinary because the certified group leader may be a nurse, activities director, social worker, or even a volunteer or family member. Sessions should be held consistently not only to reinforce trust and promote bonding but also to attain the goals of the therapy sessions. One of the limitations to its multidisciplinary approach is that group leaders may wear many hats, so providers must prioritize the scheduling of remotivation therapy sessions on patient care plans.

Following the theory component of the course, each remotivator conducts a practicum in his or her own facility. Students of remotivation therapy receive direct supervision from the instructor during the practicum and become certified at the twelfth session if their techniques are appropriate, sessions have been held consistently, patient progress reports have been documented, and twelve plans have been submitted to the instructor for review.

Satisfactory completion of the basic course earns certification from the National Remotivation Therapy Organization, Inc. Renewal is based on (1) membership in good standing of NRTO, (2) completion of fifteen hours of continuing education focused on group work, and (3) psychosocial rehabilitation or other related topics that would increase understanding and skill as a remotivation therapist (Bierma, 1998).

Following basic certification and completion of at least twenty-four remotivation sessions, the remotivator is eligible to enroll in an advanced remotivation therapy course. The advanced five-step remotivation process encourages flexibility in application and teaches remotivators skills necessary to work with the most regressed as well as with the highest functioning people. There is no formal advanced practicum required. Advanced certification is awarded at the completion of the four-day advanced classroom-based course.

The National Remotivation Therapy Organization, Inc. maintains the standards and guidelines for remotivation in the United States. It employs an executive director and is supported by a seven-member executive board and state representatives who complete the board of directors. Several states have local councils that are chapters of the national organization.

NRTO is open to all persons interested in remotivation therapy. The organization membership provides a quarterly newsletter, opportunity to attend and participate in the annual national remotivation therapy institute, voting privileges in elections, and the opportunity to hold office as a member of the board of directors (Robinson, 1967).

As an incorporated, nonprofit organization, NRTO is eligible to request and receive grants to fund training. The organization's newsletter and Web page generate much interest in communicating information to current and potential remotivators nationally and internationally. Remotivators are encouraged to write and publish their views and experiences; this helps establish a solid support system for all remotivators in various settings and organizations.

Efforts are being made to have remotivation therapy reimbursable by insurers to those facilities that have active remotivation programs. Current fiscal problems in health care have delayed this process, though some health care programs have made promising breakthroughs.

Remotivation therapy has become an integral part of patient care plans in a wide variety of settings. What started out as group therapy sessions in a psychiatric setting has expanded into a therapeutic modality effective in geriatric long-term and day care settings, social clubs, group homes for deinstitutionalized persons, substance abuse centers, prisons, and most recently, in facilities that provide programs for patients with Alzheimer's or Huntington's disease.

Over the years remotivation therapy has enjoyed the support of professionals in different disciplines. Their perspectives add further dimensions to the official definition of remotivation therapy. In 1969, Dr. Arthur Stillman, then clinical director at South Florida State Hospital, wrote an article titled "Let's Look at Remotivation." His comments addressed the group process used in remotivation therapy as supportive, re-educational, and reconstructive.

In the early 1980s, speech pathologist Jean Wicklund's (1981) position paper titled "Motivational Change in the Aging Adult" suggested that appropriate implementation of remotivation therapy increases clients' communication skills and increases interest in their immediate surroundings.

Fred Watson, president of the Georgia Nursing Home Association, has advocated for Georgia's elderly since 1953. In a letter written in 1991 to the president of the National Remotivation Therapy Organization Watson advocated for new federal regulations that would establish remotivation programs to help residents improve mental and social skills and achieve their potential.

REFERENCES

Bierma, J. (1998). *Remotivation Group Therapy: Handbook for the Basic Course.* York Harbor, ME: NRTO, Inc.

Mental Hospital Services (1956). *Remotivation Technique: Some Basic Facts.* American Psychiatric Association and Smith Kline & French Laboratories (updated from original manual by Alice M. Robinson, 1956).

Robinson, A. (1967). *Remotivation Technique.* Philadelphia, PA: Smith Kline & French.

Stillman, A. (1969). Let's Look at Remotivation. South Florida State Hospital, unpublished paper.

Wicklund, J. (1981). Remotivation: Motivational Change in the Aging Adult. Georgia Nursing Home Association, unpublished paper.

Chapter 4

Advanced Remotivation Therapy

James Siberski

OVERVIEW

Advanced remotivation therapy, like basic remotivation therapy, is a simple group therapy that utilizes the five original steps which have their roots in Dorothy Hoskins Smith's original conception of remotivation therapy. The aim of the original five basic steps is to help the patient relate to and communicate with others. Individuals trained in basic remotivation can graduate to advanced remotivation therapy after having completed a suitable number of basic sessions to gain the experience necessary to conduct the advanced sessions. In the advanced sessions, the five steps of the original remotivation therapy can be structured a bit differently (Bierma, 1998). This will be addressed later in this chapter. In advanced, the aim is to motivate the patient's interest in the affairs of everyday living. This will, in turn, help the patient cope with changes in social conditions, developments, and trends in society; the older patient may simply remain engaged and active in society. It may motivate patients by providing pleasant associations and stimuli helping them develop the desire to return to society and participate in community activities (Wilson and Kneisl, 1998).

The definition of *advanced remotivation* is a simple group therapy where the content is of an objective or subjective nature, and the therapist always remains objective. It deals objectively with both wounded and unwounded areas of the patient's personality and helps people to think about reality in relation to themselves. The five-step technique is utilized along with simulation exercises, value search sessions, and advanced word clarification/flight of idea poetry sessions. Additional training after basic remotivation training is required to learn advanced remotivation and to become a certified advanced remotivation therapist.

The advanced remotivation therapist needs to learn how to remain objective when dealing with a subjective topic, and when discussing a wounded area of a patient's personality. The remotivation therapist, doing advanced remotivation, would never "psychologize" by probing, providing interpretations to patient's statements, or confronting the patient. These techniques, as well as other psychotherapeutic group techniques, would be utilized by individuals trained in more advanced group therapy techniques.

The value of advanced remotivation for patients is that these sessions can, depending upon the patient's functional level, address the needs of high-functioning groups, where basic remotivation would tend to be more elementary. These sessions, in addition, can challenge the patient who has successfully completed basic remotivation. It can reinvigorate the patient who becomes bored in basic sessions. Older patients can easily reminisce through the advanced session, and advanced remotivation can provide a structure for a therapist to follow up with health-teaching groups.

The health-teaching advanced remotivation sessions have been used successfully in various treatment settings including prisons (Siberski, 1998). In advanced remotivation sessions with health-teaching objectives, participants are allowed to gain basic knowledge about specific health care situations or illnesses.

If the participant is experiencing the illness, the learning is of a subjective nature; if the participant is not experiencing the illness, then it is informative and objective. In both cases the participant gains objective, basic information that can be utilized in the future, perhaps in more advanced therapy situations.

In summary, the values of advanced remotivation are to challenge the bored, meet the needs of the high functioning, provide a platform for reminiscence, and teach and continue the work started in basic remotivation.

A wide variety of topics can be utilized in advanced sessions; they range from death and dying, to religious or political issues. Topics do not have to be subjective to be considered advanced. Advanced sessions can include pleasant reminiscing and/or health-teaching sessions (Varcarolis, 1998). In reminiscing sessions, the patient may start to reminisce about a wounded area. This will be permissible in advanced sessions, provided that the therapist remains objective and does not criticize, attach values, or attempt to interpret the memory. In *education* sessions (which are different from health-teaching sessions), the answers the patients give to the therapist need to be correct. The therapist, therefore, would focus on the right answer, as opposed to basic remotivation, where the therapist would accept any response given by the patient. Here, the therapist would correct the patient since accuracy is important in educational advanced remotivation sessions. Some examples of *basic* and *advanced* sessions are as follows:

Basic remotivation	Advanced remotivation
Basic diversional sessions	Upgraded sessions
[objective]	[subjective]
Activities of daily living sessions	Value judgment sessions
Sequential remotivation	Simulation sessions
Active games	Patient government sessions
	Reminiscing sessions

Remotivation therapists need to be trained in and conduct numerous basic remotivation therapy sessions before moving on to advanced remotivation therapy. The same is true for the participants/patients that the remotivation therapist would be treating. A group of patients should not sit down on the first day of remotivation therapy and discuss death and dying issues. Rather, a group should evolve through basic remotivation therapy where they can develop the abilities and skills to handle more progressive topics before starting them in advanced. Once the group is ready for advanced remotivation therapy, the therapist needs to choose the type of session carefully since the individuals will be challenged, perhaps for the first time in a long time, to deal with subjective matter.

There are various types of *advanced remotivation* sessions. They all utilize the five steps of basic remotivation with some requiring variations to some of the steps.

Step 1 is always the climate of acceptance in both basic and advanced remotivation sessions.

Step 2, in advanced remotivation, is when an activity is set up; the group can be warmed up in a verbal sense while being prepared for subsequent steps. It can also be used as a plain step 2 in basic remotivation therapy. Everyone in the group during step 2 should be encouraged to participate either nonverbally or, ideally, verbally. Step 2 should not be a demanding step.

Step 3 is a discussing, planning, and/or performing step in advanced, depending on the type of session you are conducting. This will be explained in detail later.

Step 4 always involves some type of work. It is the *action* of the session. The exception is in the reminiscing group, where step 4 defines an emotion of the topic related to the discussion.

Step 5 is always the traditional climate of appreciation.

MODELS FOR ADVANCED REMOTIVATION THERAPY

In the following paragraphs, several advanced remotivation sessions will be presented. The reader should refer to the appendix to gain a complete understanding of the structure of the advanced session under discussion.

In traditional advanced remotivation, various topics can be discussed ranging from hate, anger, fear, and failure to joy and patriotism. This type of advanced session encourages the patient to discuss subjective topics. The session follows the basic remotivation structure, with the main difference being that the topic under discussion is subjective.

The next advanced session is the *group project* session. An example of a *group project* would be "making a video." The patients are encouraged to work together, to support one another's work roles, and to produce an end product. This end product will endure even after the patient is discharged or the group is completed. Such products are informational videos, word newspapers, and community service projects, such as planting trees.

The next type of session is a *simulation* session. The patients, in *simulation* sessions, can try out different roles and discuss what they learned from the roles in a group format. Patients are coaxed into providing constructive feedback to peers in a limited fashion. Less-than-perfect results are acceptable. The patient is rewarded for trying. It will be the high-level programs and therapies that will focus on insight, perfection of product, or on process issues of the group. Topics here range from simulating a job interview to ordering a meal in a restaurant to asking the doctor for a weekend pass.

The next advanced session utilizes *poems* in a manner where the participants can clarify words, engage in a session of flight of ideas, or discuss the content of the poem. Here the patient is allowed to discover personal meaning of words found in the poem, such as "calm colors" where the word *calm* would be discussed from a personal point of view. Another example would be "exciting colors" where the participants would discuss what the word *exciting* means. It allows patients to think and explore different thoughts in depth. The depth of the exploration comes from drawing in the entire group. This type of session is valuable for patients still having difficulty staying on one topic. It allows patient groups to seek the meaning of a poem, a word, or a paragraph. In advanced remotivation, we can use subjective poetry or we can continue, as we would in basic, to use objective poetry and simply clarify the various words found throughout the poem.

Patient government is yet another form of advanced remotivation. This session is excellent for patient meetings since it provides a structure to conduct a meeting. It allows the patient to continue to voice opinions, take stands on issues, or undertake roles such as voter, good citizen, etc.

The *value search* or *value judgment* session allows the patients to begin to examine how they feel about issues in a safe milieu. Patients are not criticized no matter what side of the issue they choose to take or how outlandish their opinions might be. Patients are encouraged to think about the issue being discussed through a value search session and are encouraged to view the other side of the issue. Value search sessions can include forced-choice questions, such as, "Do you like *x* or *y*?" The patients can then think about the response that they render.

Last, *reminiscing* sessions provide typically older patients, including the cognitively impaired or demented and the mentally ill (such as schizophrenics), with a structure with which to reconstruct their memories (Siberski, 1998). Dr. Robert Butler said that life review was a normal development occurrence that all elderly engaged in as they approach death (Butler, 1981). For patients to conduct private life reviews, they must reminisce. The *reminiscing* advanced remotivation session provides the therapist with a format to discover the memories, develop the memories, and to define an emotion attached to the memory. The session would consist of a series of step 2 questions such as "What was your favorite toy when you were young?" "What type of stove did your mother have in her kitchen?" "When was the first time you went fishing?"

Then, in step 3, one by one, these memories would be developed using the who, what, where, when type of questions. "Who gave you your first toy?" "Where did you keep it?" "When did you play with it?" "Who did you play with when you had your toy?" The memory would be developed at this point.

In step 4 we would take the same topic and ask, "How did you feel when you were playing with this toy?" "Did you enjoy playing with this toy?" "What were some of your emotions that you remember such as laughter, etc.?" Having completed step 4, we would then return to the next discovered memory—"What type of stove did you have in your kitchen?"—and do a step 3 and a step 4. This would be completed on all discovered memories. We would conclude with a traditional step 5. The patients or participants in the group would now have three memories from which they could, if they chose, conduct a life review.

Looking at Outcomes

The by-products of the sessions discussed are as follows:

1. Learning from members: information exchange. *Patients might discuss what challenges they would face upon discharge.*
2. Trying out new group roles: role-playing. *A group member can become a teacher (role) or an organizer (role) in an advanced session.*
3. Tolerating subjective topics, such as divorce.
4. Preparing for higher level programming. *Members will become comfortable with subjective topics in advanced remotivation and will be able to move to insight-oriented groups.*
5. Opportunities to experience the curative factors of group therapy as defined by Irving Yalom, i.e., universality, altruism, and group cohesiveness, to mention but three (Yalom, 1983).
6. Problem solving can be developed by using problem-solving exercises in group.
7. Begin to look at values of others using value search sessions.

THE ADVANCED REMOTIVATION THERAPIST

The advanced remotivation therapist must tend to several tasks.

- Encourage participation and verbalization.
- Protect the patient if others in the group fail to understand the patient's point of view.
- Prepare session topics and guideposts ahead of time.
- Provide, through the five steps, the structure that patients need to conduct subjective groups.
- Remain accepting and neutral. *The advanced remotivation therapist never takes sides.*
- Validate, when asked, by a member or the group. *The advanced remotivation therapist might respond to the group by saying, "Yes, the group does seem to favor longer mealtimes."*
- Remain objective at all times.
- Allow all group members to participate. Do not cut off discussion or allow someone to be cut off by a group member because of value clashes.
- Do not "psychologize" at any time during the session. Do not seek values, probe for a deeper meaning, or challenge a statement.

SUMMARY

All therapists, having completed the training, will be reminded that advanced remotivation is not a cure; rather, it prepares patients for higher level programming or therapy. Advanced remotivation therapists do not focus on developing insights, correcting illogical thoughts, or resolving crises. Advanced sessions extend the benefits of a basic remotivation session to topics that are subjective in some manner.

Before patients can begin to deal with subjective material, they must be able to discuss the material. In advanced remotivation, the subjective material is discussed within the climate of acceptance. This means that the advanced remotivation therapist does not challenge the patients' statements, interpret meaning into what has been said, or attempt to revalue any information the patient has provided. The therapist accepts the patients' words, actions, and behaviors. The patient will become comfortable discussing the subjective material and will be better prepared to advance to insight-oriented and cognitive-restructuring groups.

APPENDIX: STEPS IN THE REMOTIVATION PROCESS

Advanced Remotivation

1. Traditional Advanced (Examples: topics such as hate, anger, fear, failure, joy, reverence, and patriotism)
   I. Climate of acceptance
   II. Lead up to the subjective topic
   III. Discussion of subjective topic
   IV. Work involved with the subjective topic
   V. Climate of appreciation
2. Group Project (Example: making a video)
   I. Climate of acceptance
   II. Discussion; getting to know members of group
   III. 5 W's (planning). Who has what role? Where will the work be done? What equipment is required? When does the work occur? Where are we making the video?
   IV. Doing the work
   V. Climate of appreciation
3. Simulation (Example: getting a job)
   I. Climate of acceptance
   II. Leading up to the exercise
   III. Introduction to exercise—who has what role, where simulation is taking place, and what is the desired learning outcome
   IV. The actual work of doing the simulation and subsequent discussion
   V. Climate of appreciation
4. Poem (Example of ideas, work clarification, discussion of content)
   I. Climate of acceptance
   II, III, IV. All three steps are contained within the poem
   V. Climate of appreciation
5. Patient Government
   I. Climate of acceptance
   II. Roll call
   III. Agenda items and discussion
   IV. Voting
   V. Climate of appreciation

6. Reminiscing Session
    I. Climate of acceptance
    II. Discover the memory
    III. Develop the memory
    IV. Define an emotion of the memory
    V. Climate of appreciation
7. Value Judgment (i.e., game methodology)
    I. Climate of acceptance
    II. Setup of game, rules, etc.
    III. Exercise
    IV. Work = learning
    V. Climate of appreciation

Traditional Advanced Remotivation

I. Climate of acceptance
II. The following questions might be used to stimulate discussion:
   • What is the silliest thing you have ever done?
   • What is the dumbest thing you have ever done?
   • What is the worst thing you have ever bought?
   • What is one choice you had to make today?
III. The following scenarios might be used to stimulate discussion:
   • Your house catches fire. You have saved your family and pets, and you can save one more thing. What will that be?
   • If you could use a voodoo doll to hurt anyone you chose, would you?
   • Would you prefer to be blind or deaf?
   • You finish a meal and the check comes. You notice that you were not charged for one expensive item. Do you tell the waitress?
   • You are given a million dollars to give to charity. To whom do you give it?
IV. The following questions might be used to stimulate discussion:
   • How do you make choices?
   • What are the first, second, third, steps?
   • Is it hard work for you?
   • Do you use anything besides your brain to make choices?
V. Climate of appreciation

Reminiscing Session

I. Climate of acceptance
II. The following questions might be used to stimulate discussion:
   • What is the first toy you can remember?
   • What kind of stove did your mother cook on?
   • What was your first car?

III. The following are possible follow-up questions to those posed previously:

Toy:
- Who gave you this toy?
- Where did you play with the toy?
- When did you play with the toy?
- What was your favorite thing about the toy?

Stove:
- What did your mother cook on the stove?
- What did it smell like when she cooked on the stove?
- When did your mother show you how to use the stove?

Car:
- What color was the car?
- Where did you drive in the car?
- Where did you park the car?
- When did you sell the car?

IV. The following subjective questions might help to continue discussion around the topic areas of toys, stoves, and cars:

Toy:
- How did you feel when you played with the toy?
- Did you ever get mad at the toy?
- How did you feel when you shared the toy?

Stove:
- Do you remember how you felt when you helped your mother cook?
- How did you feel when you used the stove for the first time?

Car:
- Were you scared when you took your driving test?
- How did you feel after you waxed your car?
- How did you feel the first time you drove in the snow?

V. Climate of appreciation

Simulation Session

I. Climate of acceptance
II. The following subjective questions might help to continue discussion:
- How should you dress for a job interview?
- What documents should you take to an interview?
- Should you arrive early?
- Who do you think you would meet first?

III. The following role-play scenario might help to continue discussion:
- Who wants to be the secretary?
- Who wants to be the job seeker?
- Who wants to be the personnel manager?
- Who will volunteer to set up the room?
- What are some questions one might be asked?
- "Let's give it a try!"

IV. Execute and evaluate the role-play (What did they learn?)

V. Climate of appreciation

REFERENCES

Bierma, J. (1998). *Remotivation group therapy: Handbook for the basic course.* York Harbor, ME: NRTO, Inc.

Butler, R.N. (1981). The life review: An unrecognized bonanza. *International Journal of Aging and Human Development,* 12(1): 35-38.

Siberski, J. (1998). Have you tried remotivation therapy lately? *Activity Director Guide* 25(6): 1-2.

Varcarolis, E. (1998). *Foundations of Psychiatric Mental Health,* Fifth Edition. Reading, MA: Addison-Wesley Publishing Company, Inc.

Wilson, H.S. and Kneisl, C.R. (1998). *Psychiatric Nursing,* Fifth Edition. Reading, MA: Addison-Wesley Publishing Company, Inc.

Yalom, I. (1983). *Inpatient Group Psychotherapy.* New York: Basic Books, Inc.

Chapter 5

All the Possibilities

Michael L. Stotts

About forty years ago, Robert S. Garber wrote in "A Psychiatric View of Remotivation" why remotivation works. At the time, he was chair of the American Psychiatric Association's Remotivation Project Advisory Committee. Now, at the beginning of the twenty-first century, remotivation continues to work in the hands of remotivators who understand and know the applications.

You have to wonder why this "best kept secret" is not well known; why it has not been embraced by health professionals; why it has not caught the eye of state and federal surveyors and other standard-setting officials. Why was it abandoned by the American Psychiatric Association after the Association's years of support and direct involvement as a principal proponent?

In this anthology of remotivation some answers to these questions are revealed and explored. The general intention here is to inform, even convince, the reader that remotivation can work with many different populations. It can work in a variety of settings. It can be used in the hands of any health professional or technician. It is appropriate for use with very sick people; it is effective with the well. Some remotivators use it in their families; others frequently cite its benefits in one-to-one encounters. Most important, it is designed to be used in groups. This discussion will focus on remotivation with groups in many different settings.

Not all of the special populations are described here, nor are all of the multiple settings where remotivation is currently used. Instead, this voluntary writing effort by very dedicated remotivators usually reflects direct experience with a special population or a unique setting. The exceptions are obvious given the chapter titles.

Two special populations housed in very special settings are noteworthy because the authors can also be read in juried publications. The *Journal of Neuroscience Nursing* published Flo Sullivan's work with colleagues from Harvard Medical School and Massachusetts General Hospital. Their research focused exclusively on six patients with Huntington's disease at a single location. Similarly, James Siberski published the results of his experiment with psychiatrically impaired inmates in a maximum security prison in *The Journal of Offender Rehabilitation.* These hallmark studies are the first documented research on remotivation therapy effectiveness. Until now, only anecdotal evidence had been cited; no clinical studies had been undertaken until the late 1990s.

Several threads are shared by successful remotivation therapy programs. These commonly held objectives could be characterized as principles that foster remotivation therapy as an integral component of the patient care program. Citing the two previous examples (Sullivan, 2001; Siberski, 2001), the offender program built in the principles *before* the activity therapy program began. The Huntington's disease remotivation program *gradually* took on the principles essential for success.

These principles include support by administration, adequate funding, public relations impact, interdisciplinary approach, acknowledgment of a remotivation program leader, research on remotivation therapy, and remotivation relationships with other institutions.

SUPPORT PRINCIPLES FOR REMOTIVATION THERAPY IMPLEMENTATION

Administrative Support

There are great differences between solid, informed support by administration and tacit support. Remotivation therapy should have a place at the planning table and should not be simply an extension of another discipline, part of an activity program, for example. Administrators should know why the remotivation program exists and generally how it contributes to patient health. Administrators should be invited to witness, if not participate, in remotivation sessions.

Adequate Funding

Remotivation should have line-item status in the operations budget of the core program. It should not be riding on the coattails of another component of the institution's budget, e.g., activities. It could well have a one-fourth to three-fourths allocation time for a staff remotivation therapist. Remotivation cannot survive if a new administrator never sees remotivation identified in the institution's budget.

Public Relations Impact

In the Brethren Home in Mechanicsburg, Pennsylvania, and in the National Lutheran Home in Rockville, Maryland, the public relations impact is well understood by administrators and members of the health team. Remotivation therapy reinvigorates and adds vitality to a person, makes the client or patient more interesting, improves communication, and contributes measurably to more positive client or patient encounters. Families, staff, and members of the larger community recognize the vast differences between isolated, alienated, or noncompliant patients and those who are more actively involved as a result of their participation in remotivation sessions. These vast differences are easy to see by anyone who takes the trouble to look.

Interdisciplinary Approach

Despite all that has been written about the merits of an interdisciplinary approach to care, there are detractors and nonbelievers. The team approach has been universally accepted, particularly in management books and articles and similarly applauded in the health administration literature. However, we need only look at the corporate scandals, e.g., Enron, to realize that decision making in so many entities remains solely at or near the top. On the other hand, ample evidence supports success when decision making is shared, consensus is not viewed as intractable, and trust among staff members is the order of the day. The remotivation therapist must be a member of the patient care team, the planning process, and a contributor to interdisciplinary delivery of services.

Acknowledgment of a Remotivation Leader

The care program leadership must recognize a spokesperson for remotivation therapy. This is the person who attends patient care conferences, trains others to become remotivation therapists, and provides the minimal resource to staff, administration, and the community on all matters dealing with remotivation and patient or client progress. The job description reflects an in-depth understanding of remotivation. The person should be certified at the advanced or instructor levels by the National Remotivation Therapy Organization.

Research on Remotivation

Where remotivation therapy is practiced, intramural and/or extramural research should also be evident. Every remotivator can tell you stories of changes brought by remotivation sessions. Not always are the case studies documented. In other situations, the remotivator has done impact evaluation studies and, in rare cases, controlled research has been the academic partner of remotivation therapy practice.

Remotivation Relationships with Other Institutions

The public has become increasingly aware of the vast differences between a teaching hospital and a hospital that does not own that designation. Television, through programs such as *ER* and *St. Elsewhere,* features the importance of relationships particularly with academic institutions. Reports from successful remotivation programs demonstrate great advantages to all participants. Where remotivation concepts can be shared with other programs that emphasize high quality of care standards, remotivation is more likely to be adopted by the other partners. The relationships can include research partnerships, liaisons with sister health delivery programs, or community-based education centers such as area health education centers (Bierma, 1998; Grozier, 2001, personal communication).

The seven principles presented here are a summary of observations made by the author about existing successful programs and about the remotivators whose unflagging optimism created very fine models. Some of these models are described in this chapter; other models are described elsewhere in this anthology. Other fine models exist in the United States, Canada, and Australia that are not documented here.

As a result of a series of personal communications with several remotivators, three models were selected for inclusion here because of their unique character.

THREE SAMPLES
OF REMOTIVATION THERAPY MODELS

Model I: Adele-Joan Warnke's Volunteer and Independent Living Programs

Your perception of my uniqueness concerning remotivation therapy is correct, but [it] is a little more than my volunteer program. I am also the activities director for the independent living program at the home, and I use it there also.

Remotivation therapy works well in my programs as my volunteers are trained in the therapy and use it with resident groups every week. At present we have eight to ten therapy groups a week and many one-to-one therapy sessions in the residents' rooms.

I use it myself in my independent living programs. Believe it or not, I find that my training enters into how I do things even with the staff (in-services) and my volunteers (recognition programs, etc.).

What would it take to duplicate my model elsewhere? Enough trained people; an administration that will go along with the program and let you educate new volunteers as they come into your program; therapists that are willing to try new ideas with the therapy, like doing one-to-ones.

I think every group you have must be handled differently. You must know your group well and know what they are capable of doing. Our groups with the Alzheimer's residents must be led in a manner that takes into consideration the Alzheimer's residents' limitations: shorter groups, more visuals, being able, [to] in a quiet, slow way bring them back to the target of the discussion. In some groups eye contact is all you will receive and an answer is something that doesn't come easily. Each remotivator has to be hand picked to be able to lead each group. All personalities aren't perfect for every group.

Our home residents on the different floor levels must have different levels of remotivation adapted to what they can handle in the group and what their needs are. We have ladies' and mens' groups and, of course, mixed groups.

I find remotivation therapy a wonderful tool that can be adapted in many ways for use in the community that you are serving.

Adele-Joan Warnke, ADC, CrmT II, CVM
Director of Volunteer Services and ILP Director of Activities,
National Lutheran Home for the Aged, Rockville, Maryland

Model II: John R. Bierma's Teaching and Promoting Remotivation in an Area Health Education Center

The uniqueness of remotivation therapy (medical settings) or remotivation technique (educational settings) makes teaching and promoting it a challenge. The interdisciplinary or multidisciplinary nature of remotivation prevents an individual professional discipline from claiming it as their exclusive area of practice. There have been movements by remotivators to create a discipline of remotivation therapy, like physical therapy or recreational therapy. These efforts usually die out when people realize that the efforts undermine the unique cross-discipline nature of remotivation. In addition to remotivation being interdisciplinary, it is also unique in that paraprofessionals and volunteers can practice it (within the state laws and/or the policies of the agency/facility) with proper supervision. People continually try to make remotivation into a cure of some disease(s). This is directly contrary to the definition of remotivation, which states that it focuses on the healthy, unwounded aspects of the personality. Remotivation can be a part of caring for someone just as patient education is part of good care. But education does not cure disease by itself.

In light of the above, professional disciplines such as nursing, recreational therapy, social work, and psychiatry have not widely taught remotivation as a skill within their disciplines because it cannot be used to corner the market for them in the health care funding stream. This poses the question of who could and will teach and promote remotivation if professional disciplines and the degree programs at colleges and universities that are accredited by those professional groups will not teach it. To answer this question, you must look for organizations or advocacy groups that seek to promote the health of the populations without regard to their pocketbook or professional turf. One such organization is an area health education center (AHEC).

Mission

The mission of the area health education center's program is to improve the supply and distribution of health care professionals, with an emphasis on primary care, through community/academic educational partnerships, to increase access to quality health care.

I have worked for eighteen years in AHEC centers in North Carolina and in Mississippi. During this period, I have had the opportunity to present remotivation as a skill to licensed health care professionals who could bill insurance companies, Medicaid and Medicare, for remotivation when provided within their scope of professional practice. I have also offered it to paraprofessionals and volunteers as skills that they could use in their relations with the elderly, adolescents, young children, the developmentally disabled, the mentally ill, and substance abusers. I have offered it as a skill to teachers in public schools who need to learn to motivate troubled students who are in in-school suspension.

The mission of AHEC allowed me to do this without conflict with my profession or from work demands that were of a higher priority. Many nurses, social workers, and activity professionals are certified to teach others in remotivation skills, but their work demands prevent them from devoting significant time to it. Their jobs do not put them in settings or relationships with agencies and community groups to easily promote remotivation. An AHEC staff person is continually assessing the needs of his or her community, health care providers, and facilities. Having remotivation as an individual skill to offer health professionals, and as a program for a facility to develop, greatly enhances the value of an AHEC to its community. It is a skill that truly brings people together in client- or patient-focused care and education.

All AHEC centers are affiliated with academic medical centers. Many of the AHEC staff, as I have, hold faculty appointments at the medical schools as instructors or adjunct assistant professors. This lends a degree of authority and quality assurance to remotivation training when it is supported by the credibility of the university system.

Remotivation and Dorothy Hoskins Smith, the developer of remotivation, are ahead of their time in concept and action. As information explodes and professional groups fight to maintain turf within this constantly changing landscape of our culture, remotivation will be a leader in the interdisciplinary delivery of health care and in the quality delivery of education of adults and children.

AHEC centers are ideal places for remotivation to be promoted in local communities in partnership with the health care providers and teachers in that community. AHEC centers can have their own staffs trained as certified remotivation instructors or they can sponsor existing remotivation instructors from around the country to teach remotivation workshops in their local communities.

John R. Bierma, MA, CRmT, Instructor II,
and Former Executive Director,
Delta Area Health Education Center, Greenville, Mississippi

Model III: James Siberski's Remotivation in a State Mental Health Hospital

Danville State Hospital in Danville, Pennsylvania, models itself on those state mental health institutions that had highly active remotivation programs in the late 1960s and the 1970s. Danville retained its remotivation therapy program during the great waves of transferring hundreds of patients to community nursing homes. In addition, it has assumed a leadership role by continuing to train personnel in remotivation from the larger health community (approximately a 100-mile radius, including prisons). Several reasons account for the success of this model:

- remotivation plays a central role;
- training of staff is a high priority;
- management creates an expectation of success among staff;
- staff members are given the time to prepare and present;
- remotivation is perceived to actually transmit skills, confidence, and motivation for patients to take the next higher step to more advanced therapy;
- an in-house training program is less expensive than any other; and
- training in remotivation extends beyond the hospital into the community.

As the director of staff development at Danville, I have strong clinical skills that allow me to be conversant with medical staff and with the superintendent's office. In a sense, my affiliation with Philadelphia State Hospital, where I trained in remotivation, became a bridge to the original and highly successful model for remotivation training. My position gives me the ability to influence training policy and, therefore, to feature remotivation in all training in the hospital. Because of our success at Danville, the hospitals at Wernersville, Harrisburg, Clarks Summit, and others have requested training by us in remotivation therapy. We train the trainers and assist other staff development officers to recreate our model in their own hospital communities.

The chief executive officer, to whom I report directly, utilizes my expertise as we train in nursing homes, personal care homes, hospitals both public and private, community mental health programs, and prisons. Through training and presentations that I do privately, these activities generate additional interest in remotivation therapy. In a sense, Danville is a regional center (east central Pennsylvania) for remotivation training.

In my position I am responsible for three clinical and nonclinical training staff members. Over the years, I have developed an unusually strong position where I am able to direct the clinical training course for the hospital which in turn largely translates into the clinical program. I chair many committees, including the Collaborative Practice Committee. This committee evaluates, assesses, and sets the course for therapy throughout the hospital. We use the biopsychosocial-spiritual model in all programs.

Remotivation works at Danville because of our results-oriented training program. It also achieves our goals because it

- does not require advanced group skills on the part of patients;
- is not psychologically intrusive and therefore [is] "safe";
- requires patients to use numerous cognitive skills;
- utilizes only patients' strengths; and
- avoids dwelling on negatives and symptoms of deficits.

James Siberski, MS CrmT, Instructor II
Director of Staff Development, Danville (Pennsylvania) State Hospital

CHALLENGES FOR REMOTIVATORS

Perhaps there are more, but here are four challenges for remotivators and the National Remotivation Therapy Organization (NRTO) that serves them. These coincide with the principles discussed previously; however, the issues are national and organizational, and at the present time, largely recognized by the leadership of NRTO.

Publicity

Clearly, remotivation therapy must be expanded beyond the ten to twelve states where it is known. To use Massachusetts as an example, remotivation efforts are well organized because of several dedicated people. Not all states have leaders who sponsor training, hold workshops, network among health professionals, and demonstrate and promote remotivation therapy.

Research

Closely allied with extending the use of remotivation is conducting new research and publicizing its effectiveness in journals, books, and news accounts. This is no simple task. It will require ingenuity and perseverance by individuals who will make this their personal priority. It may happen with help from partners in the health disciplines or in other associations, e.g., Alzheimer's Association, AARP, etc. NRTO is taking responsibility by urging its members to publish research about remotivation.

Collaboration

Remotivation thrived under the auspices of the American Psychiatric Association in its earliest days. Many leaders in psychiatry throughly believed in remotivation technique and, as a consequence, genuinely desired to support this "new" therapy in its formative years. Since that time, NRTO has unsuccessfully tried to liaison with several national organizations. At present, only the Canadian and Australian remotivation organizations have affiliations with NRTO. New affiliations must be found with organizations that share NRTO's mission and goals.

Availability of Training

Training in remotivation therapy exists in about six to nine locations, usually in the state where a certified instructor lives and works. Some exceptions to this model have provided greater opportunities to serve a wider geographical area. These exceptional models show great promise and should be encouraged. Examples include distance learning opportunities over the Internet, regional training centers, corporate sponsorships, grants that provide scholarships, and training that is sponsored as a part of a course curriculum, particularly in a community college.

SUMMARY

Where remotivation therapy is practiced by able and dedicated servants, the remotivation therapy program will produce visible results. Where remotivation therapy is practiced *without* the supports necessary for continuity and credibility, the remotivator "tilts at windmills." Where remotivation therapy is institutionalized in the care program, if the lead remotivator leaves the position or the administrator is replaced by another, remotivational therapy will continue to thrive. Where imagination, in the hands of a skillful lead remotivator, improves the capacity of remotivation therapy to contribute positives to patients' and clients' mental health, families and other patient advocates will demand appropriate support of remotivation techniques.

REFERENCES

Bierma, J. (1998). *Remotivation group therapy: Handbook for the basic course.* York Harbor, ME: NRTO, Inc.

Siberski, J. (2001). Response of psychiatrically impaired inmates to activity therapy. *Journal of Offender Rehabilitation* 33(3): 65-75.

Sullivan, F., Bird, E., Menekse, A., and Jang-Ho, J. (2001). Remotivation therapy and Huntington's disease: A path to better living. *Journal of Neuroscience Nursing* 33(3): 136-142.

Chapter 6

Evidence-Based Remotivation: An Application of Self-Determination Theory in Mental Health, Substance Abuse, and Developmental Disabilities

John R. Bierma

HISTORICAL CONTEXT

Remotivation therapy was born within the context of the mental health treatment of persons in institutions and VA hospitals after World War II. The improved functioning resulting from the application of remotivation prompted training in 135 hospitals of some 6,000 nurses and attendants. As of 1962 over 60,000 patients had participated in remotivation (McCormick, 1962). During the 1960s the American Psychiatric Association formed a remotivation advisory committee to oversee a remotivation project within its Mental Hospital Service. This project established clinical guidelines and a training manual for remotivation instruction (Garber, 1965).

INTENDED OUTCOMES OF REMOTIVATION

Dorothy Hoskins Smith described her technique of interaction with patients as remotivation. The name was intended to indicate the objective of the intervention. Therefore, the outcome of remotivation is motivation. The level of motivation in the client and in the staff would be increased as a result of the intervention. Motivation was measured by a person's voluntary, intrinsic desire to do something and perform the action without either internal or external rewards or punishments. In the most extreme cases of demotivation, patients had become mute, refusing to respond to staff with speech. When staff interacted with these unmotivated patients using remotivation techniques, the clients began to talk for the first time to staff. Also, because the patients began to respond to staff, the staff developed increased motivation to take actions with the patients.

SCIENTIFIC RESEARCH OUTCOMES

The following studies are examples of evidence that remotivation does motivate people with various kinds of disability and illness, in various kinds of living situations, and at various levels of cognitive ability.

Study #1

The first research study to determine the outcomes of remotivation was commissioned by the American Psychiatric Association. It compared patients receiving remotivation to patients in a control group on both the acute admission wards and long-term chronic wards of a psychiatric hospital. The patients in the remotivation group improved significantly more than the controls on both the acute and chronic wards in their motivation to engage in normal activities of daily living and participate in treatment. In addition, staff attitudes toward patients became more positive (Long, 1965).

Study #2

The next study was conducted in a state school for the mentally retarded. Two groups of residents diagnosed as epileptic were matched for age (59.4 years), verbal IQ (77), and years lived in the school (Kimbrell and Luck, 1966). Both groups were taught the same information. The control group was taught using a standard lecture/discussion method and the experimental group was taught using remotivation group methods. Multiple measures were used to determine outcomes. The experimental remotivation group scored significantly better on all measures compared to the control group. It scored better on content learned and on level of comprehension. It was also rated to perform better on

1. level of interest,
2. ability to respond to direct questions,
3. volunteering of information,
4. relevancy of verbal expression to content,
5. level of self-awareness,
6. level of cooperation,
7. consideration for others in the group, and
8. level of self-confidence.

Study #3

An evaluation was conducted of the outcomes of remotivation on severely retarded children at a state training school (Stermlicht, Siegel, and Deutsch, 1971). Mentally retarded children who were profoundly disabled, ages six to thirty years, were cared for by staff using remotivation. The group served as its own control group over a twelve-week period of time. The children had a mean IQ of 18.7, mean cognitive ability (CA) of 4-4, range of 1-9 to 8-6. Children participated in remotivation group sessions three times per week. The measure of motivation was the Behavior Rating Scale. The group significantly increased its level of orientation to the environment and its level of social interaction.

Study #4

This study looked at the effect of intensive remotivation on institutionalized geriatric patients in a state mental hospital (Bovey, 1971). Experimental group #1 received five group sessions of remotivation each week for six weeks. Experimental group #2 had a person simply read from a book to them five times per week for six weeks. The control group received no intervention other than routine care. Motivation was measured by the Hospital Adjustment Scale, which assessed communication and interpersonal relations, care of self, and social responsibility, and involvement in work, activities, and recreation. In addition, environmental awareness measured by the Bender-Gestalt Test and self-concept measured by the Draw-a-Person Test was assessed.

The remotivation group significantly improved on all six variables compared to the control group. The reading group did not show improvement on two of the six variables—communication and interpersonal relations and involvement in work, activities, and recreation. Any four variables in which both the remotivation group and reading group improved in comparison to the control group, the remotivation group improved significantly more than the reading group.

Study #5

Project Share was a study that assessed the effects of remotivation on residents of a home for the aged (Arje, 1973). This study design consisted of an experimental remotivation group and a control group. The study time period was twenty-one weeks and the remotivation group was held two times each week. Motivation was measured by the following:

1. Socialization Index (SI)
2. Mental Status Schedule and Geriatric Supplement (MSS-GS)
3. Philadelphia Geriatric Morale Scale (PGC)
4. Remotivation Kit Evaluation Form
5. Individual progress notes in the medical record
6. Index of Activities of Daily Living (ADL)
7. Enjoyment of group sessions
8. Reduction of restlessness on the ward
9. Interest in participating in routine activities

The remotivation group scores were significantly higher than the controls in the following areas: socialization, mental status, morale, interest, appreciation, and relations with other members of the group.

The remotivation group increased its creative activities in recreation between the first and twenty-first week. In comparison, the control group's creative activities decreased during the same time period. The remotivation group increased its engagement in competitive activities. The control group showed no change. The remotivation group improved in its conducting of activities of daily living (ADLs).

Heavy skilled care patients improved most in

1. dressing,
2. toileting,
3. transfer from bed to chair and from wheelchair to regular chair, and
4. ability to feed themselves.

Intermediate care patients improved most in bathing themselves.

Study #6

The study looked at remotivation outcomes with older geriatric patients living in a VA hospital. The people employing remotivation were elementary schoolchildren serving as volunteers in the occupational therapy department (Thralow and Watson, 1974). Two groups were formed, a control and an experimental group. The experimental group received remotivation by the schoolchildren twice a week for fourteen weeks. The research period spanned twenty weeks. Level of motivation was measured using the Nurses Observation Scale of Inpatient Evaluation (NOSIE-30) at the start of the study, at week eleven, and at four weeks after the end of remotivation sessions. The remotivation group improved significantly over the control group in

1. neatness of dress and living quarters,
2. total positive score and overall score,
3. level of interest increased, and
4. level of irritability and total negative score decreased.

At four weeks following the end of remotivation sessions, there was no significant decline in NOSIE-30 scores for the experimental group. The patients also were rated to have improved in their amount of travel, quality of their interpersonal relationships, and quality of life in the hospital.

Study #7

This study looked at the motivational effects on both staff and patients in a nursing home (Pruitt, 1976). In this study the group served as its own control group. Residents received one remotivation session per week for twelve weeks. Motivation was measured by the

- Kogan Attitude Toward Old People Scale
- Berger Self-Acceptance Scale
- Bryfield and Rothe Index of Job Satisfaction
- Remotivation Kit Evaluation
- Humanization of Patient Care Index

The patients receiving remotivation sessions increased in motivation over the course of the study. The staff that conducted remotivation with patients improved their attitudes, and level of motivation increased. In contrast, staff attitudes of registered nurses and administrators who did not conduct sessions with the patients became negative toward the patients and their motivation decreased during the time of the study.

Study #8

Another study was conducted on the outcome of remotivation in a state psychiatric hospital. This study measured the effects of remotivation on a patient group with the specific diagnosis of schizophrenia (Beal et al., 1977). The experimental design for this study was Solomon four-group design. One control group and three experimental groups were formed as follows:

Group #1 received remotivation followed by activity.
Group #2 received remotivation followed by more remotivation.
Group #3 received traditional psychodynamic group therapy.
Group #4 control received no treatment.

The measures of motivation were the rating of levels of patients' verbal expressions and patients' ability to initiate and plan an activity. Group #1, which received remotivation followed by activity, was the only group that could voluntarily plan and conduct an activity. Group #1 was most verbal, group #2 was next best, group #3 did poorly, and group #4 had the least verbal expression.

Study #9

This study looked at the motivational effects of remotivation in comparison to traditional group psychodynamic group therapy (Greenfield, 1977). A control group and two experimental groups were formed of geriatric patients in a VA hospital. Experimental group #1 experienced twelve remotivation sessions during the first four weeks and group psychotherapy during the second four weeks. Experimental group #2 experienced only group psychotherapy for the entire eight weeks. Motivation was measured using the Affect Balance Scale, Life Satisfaction Index A, Depression Adjective Checklist, Remotivation Kit Evaluation, and the Nurses Observation Scale. Each group was tested at the beginning, midpoint, and end of the time period of eight weeks. In comparison to group #2, the remotivation/psy-chotherapy group was more active at both midpoint and at the end. The remotivation/psychotherapy group was better adjusted toward life at midpoint than either the psychotherapy group or the control group.

Study #10

This study looked at the outcomes of remotivation with elderly persons who were isolated and unmotivated living in single-family homes (Harris and Bodden, 1978). Older persons who were living independently in their homes who were unwilling to travel or visit others received "individual," one-on-one remotivation sessions each week for a six-week period of time and were compared to a control group. The persons receiving remotivation significantly improved in fifteen of sixteen personality factors in their levels of motivation measured by the Personality Factor Questionnaire developed by Cattell in 1949. The remotivation groups also improved in the factors of ego strength, trust, reduced anxiety, increased extroversion, and degree of independence.

Study #11

This study is a review of literature as of 1982 on the efficacy of group work with persons diagnosed with schizophrenia in inpatient and outpatient settings (Scott and Griffith, 1982). Researchers concluded that traditional forms of psychodynamic group therapy do not produce significant outcomes with this client population, but that remotivation group sessions did improve client outcomes in the areas of social interaction when provided in an inpatient setting. The improved social interaction increased the rates of discharge to community settings.

Study #12

This thesis for a master's degree in nursing administration retro-spectively looked at documentation in progress reports on the behavior of patients/residents/clients in a state hospital, community residential facility, a psychiatric social club, and a rehabilitation program that offered remotivation (Herlihy-Chevalier, 1987). The study showed that clients improved from remotivation sessions as measured by increases in self-esteem, self-fulfillment, social functioning, and self-actualization.

Study #13

Koppel, Carnes, and Grozier (1992) studied the effects of remotivation on the length of stay of elderly on the medical wards of an acute care hospital. Results indicated that patients receiving remotivation as compared to a control group had a decreased length of stay resulting in a savings to the hospital of $1,400 per hospital admission (Koppel, Carnes, and Grozier, 1992).

RESEARCH ON MOTIVATION, SELF-DETERMINATION THEORY, AND REMOTIVATION METHODS

The previous research studies and the other chapters in this anthology of remotivation convincingly show that remotivation does motivate people to take action relative to people and things in their lives.

The nature of the motivation developed by remotivation can be characterized as intrinsic as opposed to extrinsic motivation. Intrinsic motivation, presented by Deci and Ryan (1987) in a very comprehensive study of the theories of motivation and research, is supported by current research in motivation. The theory of motivation that has resulted from recent research beginning with the work of Deci and Ryan is self-determination theory. Research developed to test the self-determination theory of motivation has shown that people will accept more responsibility for behavior change when motivated internally rather than externally (Williams et al., 1991). These studies show that people (teachers, parents, therapists, doctors) can facilitate another person's motivation to change if they give that person three things: (1) choice, (2) relevant information, and (3) acknowledgment of the person's perspective.

Remotivation, since its inception fifty years ago, has performed each of these actions because of the behavior of the remotivation therapist. These behaviors are incorporated into the open-ended questions about the topic of the remotivation session that allow the client to state his or her opinion about the topic. The remotivation therapist's acceptance of the client's opinion without judgment or comment is the acknowledgement of the client's perspective.

Further research has shown that people with higher levels of "intrinsic motivation," the kind that remotivation develops in clients, is correlated with improved performance by people of different ages, different ability levels, and with various diseases, just as with remotivation. Examples of research showing this correlation are as follows:

1. Learning disabled children with higher levels of intrinsic motivation perform better in mathematics and reading on standardized tests (Deci et al., 1992).
2. Mothers, whose behavior with their six- to seven-year-old children supported the development of intrinsic motivation, had children more willing to make choices and to engage in activity (Deci et al., 1993).
3. Three contextual factors (the behavior of persons in the environment of the client)—namely, providing a meaningful rationale, acknowledging the behaver's feeling and opinions, and conveying choice—promote the healthy internalization of rules or regulations that are owned by the client and thereby become intrinsicly motivating (Deci et al., 1994).
4. Persons in an autonomously supportive and motivating context for losing weight attended more sessions, lost more weight, and kept it off longer (Williams et al., 1996).
5. Patients who had higher levels of autonomous motivation and were prescribed medication took it for one month and were expected to continue taking it, and adhered or complied with the doctor's orders more than those who had low levels of autonomous motivation (Williams et al., 1998).
6. Patients with diabetes who perceived that their care providers were supportive of their autonomy (accepting) were more likely to conduct self-care that resulted in improved glucose control. They specifically regulated their glucose levels better, felt more able to do it, and showed clinical improvement in their Hba1c values (Williams, Freeman, and Deci, 1998).
7. Adolescents who experienced a presentation on smoking called "It's Your Choice" that was more autonomous supportive and thereby created more intrinsic motivation to either refrain from smoking or smoke less were actually more likely to refrain and smoke less. When adolescents perceived messages

about smoking as autonomy supportive (accepting), they had more motivation not to smoke, and that, in turn, predicted a decrease in their self-reports of smoking (Williams et al., 1999).

8. A study of 1,137 adult smokers found that higher levels of intrinsic motivation relative to extrinsic motivation were associated with more advanced stages of readiness to quit smoking and successful cessation at twelve-month follow up (Curry, Grothaus, and McBride, 1997).

9. This study examined client motivation as a predictor of retention and therapeutic engagement across the major types of treatment studies in the third national drug abuse treatment outcome study (DATOS). Indicators of intrinsic motivation, especially a client's readiness for treatment, were significant predictors of engagement and retention in treatment. More important, motivation was more predictive of outcome than were sociodemographic, drug abuse, and other background variables (Joe, Simpson, and Broome, 1998).

10. In a study of the functional performance of nursing home residents, only two factors, motivation (efficacy beliefs and intrinsic motivation) and lower extremity function (contractures and standing balance), predicted 81 percent of the client's variance in function (Resnick, 1998).

In this author's opinion, these cited studies strongly support remotivation and the concepts that are foundational to its efficacy as an intervention.

REFERENCES

Arje, F.B. (1973). Project Share: Reactions of residents of a home for the aged to a selected remotivation technique. *Dissertation Abstracts International,* Order No. 73(25):154.

Beal, D., Duckro, P., Elias, J., and Hecht, E. (1977). Graded group procedures for long-term regressed schizophrenics. *Journal of Nervous and Mental Disease* 164(2):102-106.

Bovey, J. (1971). The effects of intensive remotivation techniques on institutionalized geriatric mental patients in a state mental hospital. *Dissertation Abstracts International,* Order No. 72-4064, 112.

Curry, S., Grothaus, L., and McBride, C. (1997). Reasons for quitting: Intrinsic and extrinsic motivation for smoking cessation in a population-based sample of smokers. *Addictive Behaviors* 22(6):727-739.

Deci, E., Driver, R., Hotchkiss, L., Robbins, R., and Wilson, I. (1993). The relation of mothers' controlling vocalizations to children's intrinsic motivation. *Journal of Expressive Child Psychology* 55(2):151-162.

Deci, E., Eghrari, H., Patrick, B., and Leone, D. (1994). Facilitating internalization: The self-determination theory perspective. *Journal of Personal and Social Psychology* 62(1):119-142.

Deci, E., Hodges, R., Pierson, L., and Tomassone, J. (1992). Autonomy and competence as motivational factors in students with learning disabilities and emotional handicaps. *Journal of Learning Disabilities* 25(7):457-471.

Deci, E. and Ryan, R. (1987).The support of autonomy and the control of behavior. *Journal of Personal and Social Psychology* 53(6):1024-1037.

Garber, R. (1965). A psychiatrist's view of remotivation therapy. *Mental Hospitals.* American Psychiatric Association: Washington, DC.

Greenfield, D. (1977). Remotivation therapy: A test of a major assumption of the treatment of domiciled geriatric veterans. *Dissertation Abstracts International,* Order No. 77-25, 507.

Harris, J. and Bodden, J. (1978). An activity group experience for disengaged elderly persons. *Journal of Counseling Psychology* 25:325-330.

Herlihy-Chevalier, B. (1987). Remotivation therapy in the social rehabilitation of the mentally ill. Thesis, Anna Maria College, Paxton, Massachusetts.

Joe, G., Simpson, D., and Broome, K. (1998). Effects of readiness for drug abuse treatment on client retention and assessment of process. *Addiction* 93(8):117-190.

Kimbrell, D. and Luck, R. (1966). Remotivation of institutionalized epileptics. *Perceptual Motor Skills* 23:770.

Koppel, P., Carnes, E., and Grozier, E. (1992). Remotivation therapy and rehabilitative day program cost effective for the acutely ill elders. *The Gerontologist* 32(2):5.

Long, R. (1965). A study of staff and patient changes in expectancy, attitude, behavior following the introduction of remotivation techniques into the ward routine of a mental hospital. *Dissertation Abstracts International,* Order No. 66-467.

McCormick, E. (1962). They can be talked back to sanity. *Today's Health* (March), pp. 43, 44, 67-71.

Pruitt, S. (1976). The effects of remotivation on patients' attitudes and staff care of the patients. *Dissertation Abstracts International,* Order No. 76-13, 493.

Resnick B. (1998). Functional performance of older adults in a long-term care setting. *Clinical Nursing Research* 7(3):230-249.

Scott, D. and Griffith, M. (1982). The evaluation of group therapy in the treatment of schizophrenia. *Small Group Behavior* 13(3).

Stermlicht, M., Siegel, L., and Deutsch, M. (1971). Evaluations of a remotivation program with institutionalized retarded youngsters. *Training School Bulletin* 68(2):82-86.

Thralow, J. and Watson, C. (1974). Remotivation for geriatric patients using elementary school students. *American Journal of Occupational Therapy* 28(8):469-473.

Williams, G., Cox, E., Kouides, R., and Deci, E. (1999). Presenting the facts about smoking to adolescents: Effects of an autonomy-supportive style. *Archives of Pediatric and Adolescent Medicine* 153(9):959-964.

Williams, G., Freeman, Z., and Deci, E., (1998). Supporting autonomy to motivate patients with diabetes for glucose control. *Diabetes Care* 21(10):1644-1651.

Williams, G., Grow, V., Freedman, Z., Ryan, R., and Deci, E. (1996). Motivational predictors of weight loss and weight-loss maintenance. *Journal of Personal and Social Psychology* 70(1):115-126.

Williams, G., Quill, T., Deci, E., and Ryan, R. (1991). The facts concerning the recent carnival of smoking in Connecticut and elsewhere. *Annals of Internal Medicine* 115(1):59-63.

Williams, G., Rodin, G., Ryan, R., Grolnick, W., and Deci, E. (1998). Autonomous regulation and long-term medication adherence in adult outpatients. *Health Psychology* 17(3):269-276.

Chapter 7

Remotivation in Deinstitutionalization

Barbara Herlihy-Chevalier

INTRODUCTION

In the past thirty years, the census in mental health institutions has decreased from thousands to hundreds as many of the clients have been transferred from hospitals to community settings. In 1980, Dr. Donald Langsley, the 109th president of the American Psychiatric Association, reiterated the late President Kennedy's proposal for "a bold new approach" that would (1) provide for early diagnosis and continuous comprehensive care, (2) stimulate improvements in the level of care given the mentally ill in state and private institutions, and (3) provide reorientation programs in a community-centered approach whereby the mentally ill and mentally retarded could be returned to and retained in community facilities.[1] One important therapeutic regime widely used by geriatric and psychiatric health care providers was a structured form of group dynamics called remotivation therapy, which became a key modality in the deinstitutionalization process.

As preparation for deinstitutionalization, remotivation sessions were geared toward prevention or reversal of regression in clients and toward maintenance of optimal level of functioning. As further enhancement, Dr. William Petrie stated at the 1980 Institute of the National Remotivation Therapy Organization (NRTO), in Nashville, Tennessee, that a therapeutic alliance was essential because the client needed to contract to work for himself or herself.[2] Remotivation is one means of promoting this because, in working with the healthy parts of the personality, remotivation therapy enables a client to realize his or her own strengths and to focus on them. Dr. Petrie also stated that healing depends on the client's attitude, awareness, and adjustment.

In forming a support system, staff needed to seek reasons for client complaints, needed to look beyond the pathological symptoms that could be deceptive, and needed to find the strengths in clients. It was important to retain empathy and understanding as clients dealt with ambivalent feelings toward deinstitutionalization. On one hand, they were eager to leave the hospital to reenter the outside world but, on the other hand, they were frightened to think they would not be able to make it. Staff needed to lend support but not become depended upon, while clients had to learn to stand on their own two feet.

William L. Marion and Daniel A. Grabski have stated that five categories of skills were essential for community placement:

1. behavior control, which is most important,
2. self-care (dressing, grooming, toileting, eating, ambulation, care of environment),
3. social skills (including speech, orientation, and response),
4. community skills, and
5. vocation and academic skills.[3]

In attaining these skill levels, the psychosocial approach (sensory awareness, reality orientation, and remotivation) was used to increase response to the environment.

Community awareness topics led to successful deinstitutionalization as they focused on entertainment, restaurants, shopping, and housing. Field trips as follow-up to remotivation sessions fostered community utilization, independence, and adaptation. The overall deinstitutional goal at a state hospital for the mentally ill was to revitalize the patient's healthy roles through understanding, respect, touch, eye contact, reality orientation, and concrete discussion.

Typical remotivation therapy sessions were planned to increase client interest in surroundings and to promote communication and self-esteem, thereby trying to maintain an optimal level of functioning for each group member. Sessions were held in a home-like atmosphere where an expectation for more socially acceptable behavior was established.

Meal preparation and other activities of daily living were encouraged at a small cottage on hospital grounds. Small groups traveled by public transportation to the city where there were opportunities for breakfast and lunch in restaurants, as well as leisure tours. Clients needed to hold their own money and budget for bus fare, meals, and tipping. Older, less independent clients enjoyed visits to nursing homes and aftercare visits from remotivators following transfer. Clients were encouraged to take "just one step at a time" with the help of their remotivation support system.

Many benefits were realized by the caregiver, client, and facility. Successful implementation of a program stimulated the remotivators to take more interest in the clients and, at the same time, to realize more pride and accomplishment in their work. In 1978, Eleanor Flood asserted that any person, despite confusion, apathy, loneliness, depression, or dementia, could benefit from a remotivation session.[4] She also believed that remotivation therapy works because of the highly structured format consisting of five steps with emphasis on respecting the person as an adult.

Alice Robinson, who helped to develop the original remotivation manual, asserted that remotivation is a process that shows remarkable promise as a usable, economical, constructive method of patient care.[5] Dr. Donald Hammersley, former deputy medical director of the American Psychiatric Association and a member of the NRTO Advisory Board, advocated ongoing assistance by remotivators. At the 1980 Institute of NRTO, he challenged remotivators to encourage support from allies in the community and to ask legislators to remember remotivation therapy when discussing deinstitutionalization.

Adaptation from hospital to community was vital to maintain and improve the mental health of an individual and to prevent further decompensation. A state facility in Massachusetts used remotivation outcomes to develop a tool that provided a structured format for assessment in planning for deinstitutionalization.

Participants' capabilities were assessed and evaluated in areas of interest, awareness, attention span, frustration tolerance, background knowledge, reading ability, oral communication, and overall participation. Twelve session plans, which comprise a remotivation series, were developed to incorporate these areas, and small groups of clients were grouped according to level of functioning. Sessions were held consistently once or twice a week. In some cases, the first six sessions were conducted at the hospital and the remaining six sessions were conducted at the new facility.

There was liaison among remotivation and other health care disciplines such as nursing, activities, and occupational therapy. Follow-up was provided using an interdisciplinary model.

Strategies were developed for community remotivation sessions to prevent or defer reinstitutionalization, to encourage independence and the right to live with dignity in a community environment, and to provide a medium for fun and enjoyment. Paramount to every remotivator's goal was the perceived responsibility to enforce the climates of acceptance and appreciation with every client.

Community-based remotivation sessions provided a balance of structure in the unstructured settings. Topics at community residences ranged from current events and daily living activities to topics focusing on special interests and self-appreciation. Sessions preceded or were incorporated into trips and other experiences. Remotivators who had been certified in advanced therapy were also able to conduct sessions related to moods and emotions and to address controversial or problem areas. Sessions were held as part of a day program or as a form of socialization in the evening. In addition, remotivation sessions provided new insight and continuing education credits to staff who were able to promote a trusting environment by facilitating positive, friendly discussions.

Basic and advanced remotivation courses were offered to community residential staff in cooperation with the Massachusetts Department of Mental Health and the Bay State Remotivation Council, Inc. Community-based mental health centers such as the social club and adult day treatment center also became active remotivation centers and provided further rehabilitation. The most important outcomes were that people began to appreciate themselves and their potential, increasing self-esteem and socialization. They were helped to cope with change and encouraged to make new decisions.

To avoid the past disasters of deinstitutionalization, when there was a lack of planning for alternative services, remotivators and other health care providers endeavored to carry into the community the full range of treatments and services that were available at the state hospital. In 1979, John A. Talbott, a former director of the American Psychiatric Association, listed basic rules to guide future deinstitutionalization. Most notable to the remotivator was the rule which stated that "before clients are discharged, there must be an adequate number and range of community services and facilities to provide patients with treatment, care, and community support."[6] In 1981, Dr. Robert D. Miller stressed that professionals in state hospitals must continue to be involved in decision making and that familiar staff must be transitional from hospital to community.[7] Through training courses and remotivation series, remotivators were able to strengthen that liaison. Copies of remotivation progress reports were included with clients' hospital histories and aftercare orders. Dr. H. Richard Lamb stated in 1981, "If we can make long-term patients comfortable living low-energy but satisfying lives in a non-hospital environment, we have taken a great step forward in realizing the benefits expected from deinstitutionalization."[8]

A DEINSTITUTIONALIZATION MODEL

Unpublished research hypothesized that remotivation therapy is one effective method to generate improvement in the psychiatric inpatient unit, at a community residence, a social club, and a rehabilitation services center. Basic assumptions included (1) social functioning will improve with remotivation therapy, (2) there will be an increase in self-esteem and feelings of belonging, and (3) clients will experience greater self-actualization.[9] The study is an exploration into deinstitutionalization of psychiatric clients using remotivation therapy. The target population consisted of clients who had spent time on an inpatient unit before discharge to the community. Theoretical rationale focused on nursing theorist Sister Callista Roy's major emphasis on the individual's ability to adapt in situations of health and illness.[10] It also corresponded to psychologist Maslow's hierarchy of needs, which are (1) physiological, (2) safety and security, (3) belonging and social needs, (4) esteem and status, and (5) self-actualization and fulfillment.[11] A supportive model of organizational behavior was also utilized because good leadership helps remotivators to grow and to accomplish all of which they are capable.[12]

A case design was used as the plan to examine each remotivation group in the various settings in answer to evaluation questions referring to participants, goals, activities, and results. Personal interviews of these same clients asked

1. why they met each week,
2. what they did not like about the meetings,

3. what they did like about the meetings,
4. how they thought they had improved over the past year, and
5. what their ideas were for future meetings.

No comparison was made among the groups in different settings; each group was evaluated in relation to itself and in relation to the number of sessions conducted. The case design also established the existence of certain factors that could be further studied using appropriate instruments.[13] A time-series component showed collection of data about the same groups during several series or periods of time.

Nonrandom sampling provided participants who were specifically chosen as members of the various settings in need of a structured remotivation program. The sample included demographic and interview statistics of twenty-four clients involved in preplacement groups at the state hospital (1977-1981), a group of four chronically ill clients during two 12-week series (1985-1986), two clients remotivated on a one-on-one basis during three series (1985-1986), four residents at a community facility during five 12-week series (1985-1986), six members of a social club during one series (1986-1987), and one client at a rehabilitation services center during three 12-week series (1985-1986).

Threats to validity were identified, in addition to the researcher's possibly biased evaluation in favor of the program, which she coordinated, to include (1) changes in the environment while the program was in progress, (2) changes within the individuals due to medication or fluctuations in moods and emotions, (3) mortality/attrition as all participants were not able to attend all sessions because of transfers, illness, or choice, and (4) involvement in other therapies or programs such as expressive therapy, day activities programs, social events, and residential activities.

Results of the statistical analysis indicated that institutionalized and deinstitutionalized clients respond well to a structured remotivation therapy protocol, which encourages positive reinforcement and an increased autonomy. In 1977 and 1978, 120 of the elderly mentally ill transferred from the state hospital to a public health hospital for the chronically ill. The National Guard transported people by litter, by wheelchair van, and by National Guard bus. Remotivation played an important part in the transfer and support of people, most of who had spent over forty to fifty years in an inpatient hospital setting. Six preparation-for-placement sessions had been conducted focusing on clients and families, places to live, activities of daily living, and exploration of feelings. Six follow-up sessions were held at the new facility, focusing on change, safety measures, new activities, and more exploration of feelings.

Twelve men and twelve women were evaluated as to number and scoring of sessions, observations, outcomes, and recidivism. The average client age was fifty-five and average hospitalization was twenty-eight years. Eighteen clients improved in socialization and self-esteem and five increased in self-actualization. Five were transferred to the public health hospital, thirteen to nursing homes, and six to community residences. Later, six returned to the mental health hospital while eighteen were maintained in the community.

This study is significant because it shows a continuum of remotivation therapy implemented at the state hospital and expanded to applications in community settings to deinstitutionalize hospital-based clients. Remotivation therapy continued to play an integral part in the support of clients during and after the relocation protocol was implemented.

SUMMARY

In summary, remotivation therapy is a process that has shown remarkable progress as a positive, economical, and constructive method of treatment for unmotivated clients. Its multidisciplinary aspects are especially conducive because remotivators can be nurses, activities personnel, social workers, family members, or volunteers who have been certified in remotivation therapy. People must be remotivated where they are and not where others think they should be. Under the old value system, a good therapist made patients well. Endorsing the new, more realistic value system, Robert Stern and Kenneth Minhoff stated "a good therapist helps patients to retain and maintain their best level of functioning, helps them to provide for their needs, and realizes that some patients need life-long care."[14] Remotivators must be conscientious in promoting the structured technique, in setting goals and documenting outcomes, and in encouraging all clients to be as independent as possible wherever they are. Through the ongoing effort of dedicated therapists and through the therapeutic alliance of the consumers, remotivation therapy should continue to shine as a beacon of support to future deinstitutionalization efforts.

EPILOGUE

I became certified in basic remotivation therapy in 1975 and in advanced remotivation therapy in 1976. As an employee of the commonwealth of Massachusetts, I was able to implement sessions first in the public health sector and later throughout the Department of Mental Health, Region III. A certified instructor of remotivation therapy since 1977, I have taught multidisciplinary staff from psychiatric and geriatric hospitals, nursing homes, day care centers, social clubs, and, most recently, from assisted living complexes.

One of the greatest benefits of remotivation is its value to each and every remotivator as a special bond is forged with each client. It has promoted socialization and self-esteem of the caregivers as well as of the recipients.

I have enjoyed the honor and privilege of having been elected president of both the Bay State Remotivation Council, Inc. (BSRC 1980) and the National Remotivation Therapy Organization, Inc. (NRTO, 1982). I would be remiss in not acknowledging my ties with BSRC, which was the first chapter of NRTO. BSRC was founded in 1973 and incorporated as a nonprofit organization in Massachusetts in 1980. Through the pursuit and perseverance of its cofounder Agnes C. Stephen, Bay State was one of the first organizations to offer continuing education programs for its members.

As a nurse, I looked for ways to incorporate psychosocial measures with medications and treatments into total patient care. Indeed, remotivation therapy addresses the process of assessment, planning, implementation, and evaluation put forth in 1973 by the American Nurses Association as standards of nursing practice. I have been able to fulfill this process not only with the clients I have shared with but also with the students I have taught.

NOTES

1. Donald G. Langsley, "The Community Mental Health Center: Does It Treat Patients?," *Hospital Community Psychiatry,* 31, December 1980.

2. Dr. William Petrie, personal address on "Therapeutic Alliance," NRTO Institute, Nashville, TN, October 1980.

3. William L. Marion and Daniel A. Grabski, "An Assessment of a Continuing Care Program," *Hospital and Community Psychiatry,* 30, June 1979.

4. Eleanor G. Flood, Report of the Massachusetts Department of Mental Health Region III Remotivation Training Center, August 1978.

5. Alice M. Robinson, Remotivation Technique, A Manual for Use in Nursing Homes, circa 1950s.

6. John A. Talbott, "Deinstitutionalization: Avoiding Disasters of the Past," *Hospital and Community Psychiatry,* 30, September 1979.

7. Robert D. Miller, "Beyond the Old State Hospital: New Opportunities Ahead," *Hospital and Community Psychiatry,* 31, January 1981.

8. H. Richard Lamb, "What Did We Really Expect from Deinstitutionalization?," *Hospital and Community Psychiatry,* 32, February 1981.

9. Barbara Doyle Herlihy, Remotivation Therapy in the Social Rehabilitation of the Mentally Ill, a thesis project submitted in partial fulfillment of the requirements for degree of Master of Science in Nursing at Anna Maria College, Paxton, Massachusetts, 1987.

10. Julia B. George, Nursing Theories: The Base for Professional Nursing Practice. Prentice-Hall, Inc., Englewood Cliffs, NJ, 1980.

11. Keith Davis and John Newstrom, *Human Behavior at Work: Organizational Behavior,* Seventh Edition, McGraw-Hill, NJ.

12. Ibid.

13. Jacqueline Kosecoff and Arlene Fink, *Evaluation Basics: A Practitioner's Manual,* Second Printing, Thousand Oaks, CA: Sage Publications, 1984.

14. Robert Stern and Kenneth Minhoff, "Paradoxes in Programming for Chronic Patients in Community Clinic," *Hospital and Community Psychiatry,* 30, September 1979.

Chapter 8

Remotivation Therapy and Rehabilitation

Jason J. Meixsell

Remotivation therapy was originally designed to be used by psychiatric aides in mental institutions to work with their patients in a manner beyond daily custodial care (Robinson, 1967). Since that time, remotivation therapy has been used by people in several professions in a variety of settings. The professionals who make use of remotivation therapy include nurses, activity professionals, recreational therapists, social workers, occupational therapists, psychiatrists, psychologists, and more. Each professional contributes a certain aspect of his or her own profession when conducting remotivation therapy sessions.

One thing that each of these professionals has in common is that each looks to rehabilitate an individual in some manner. This rehabilitation may involve some form of physical or psychosocial rehabilitation. No matter which type of rehabilitation the professional uses, the overall goal of the sessions is to rehabilitate the patient so that he or she can live as independently as possible with the highest quality of life possible. Therefore, when these professionals make use of this technique, a rehabilitative component is added to remotivation therapy. This chapter will outline how remotivation therapy can be used by trained professionals as part of the rehabilitation program they offer.

BASIC AND ADVANCED REMOTIVATION IN PHYSICAL REHABILITATION

Basic Remotivation Therapy

Basic remotivation therapy is defined as a simple group therapy of an objective nature, designed in an effort to reach the unwounded areas of a person's personality and to get him or her thinking, once again, in the direction of reality (Meixsell, 1999; Bierma, 1998).

One of the key words in this definition is *objective*. Webster's defines the term objective as "existing outside and independent of the mind" (p. 615). Therefore, an objective topic is something that a group of people can discuss or participate in and experience in the same manner.

Bierma (1998) elaborates on the objective nature of basic remotivation by stating that sessions "focus on the reality humans share rather than the subjective reality of the self that only 'I' can experience" (p. 9). Basic remotivation therapy consists of discussions of objective topics such as cars, plants, and books.

Advanced Remotivation Therapy

Advanced remotivation therapy is defined as a simple group therapy of a subjective and objective nature designed in an effort to reach the unwounded areas of a person's personality and to get him or her thinking, once again, in the direction of reality (Siberski, October 14, 1998, personal communication). The only difference between the definitions of basic and advanced remotivation therapy is that advanced remotivation therapy adds the use of subjective topics. Advanced remotivation discusses subjective topics in an objective manner so that everyone can experience the topic, but each person will decide to use the information gained in a different way.

For example, the topic of an advanced group may be incontinence. Incontinence is a subjective topic, but it can be discussed in an objective way during the group. Although the topic of incontinence is objectively discussed, the individual group members will interpret the information that was discussed subjectively. One group member may listen to the discussion of techniques to prevent incontinence that occurred during the group session and may decide that he or she can use one of the techniques. This person learned through outsight. He or she listened to the objective discussion of a subjective topic and decided to make a change in his or her life. This type of rehabilitation is present only during advanced remotivation therapy.

The benefits of basic remotivation therapy are an increased self-esteem, increased communication, and/or increased socialization, which may be goals of a physical rehabilitation program. All of these goals can be accomplished through an objective therapy, but physical rehabilitation targets higher level skills, such as prevention of incontinence, that require the person to subjectively make a change in his or her life. Therefore, the hypothesis is that when remotivation therapy is used for the purpose of physical rehabilitation, advanced remotivation techniques are used. The following discussion will describe how remotivation therapy can be used to conduct different groups whose focus is on physical rehabilitation.

Types of Physical Rehabilitation Remotivation Groups

Self-Care Groups

The term self-care refers to several hygiene tasks that a person performs on a daily basis. Because of certain conditions, a person's performance of self-care tasks is impaired and the person needs to learn how to perform these tasks once again or learn to perform the same tasks in a different manner. The rehabilitation of these skills is something that can be conducted in both an individual and group format. From personal experience, the majority of rehabilitation programs for self-care tasks are performed with clients individually. This is due to the personal nature of many self-care tasks such as bathing and dressing. Sometimes, however, these tasks can be performed in a group format. For example, after a total hip replacement surgery a common precaution is that the person is not able to bend beyond ninety degrees. This precaution makes washing and dressing the lower body more difficult.

Part of the rehabilitation process for someone after a total hip replacement surgery is learning to use long-handled adaptive devices to assist with lower extremity bathing and dressing. The initial introduction of these devices along with education and demonstration of their use can be conducted in a group format through the use of remotivation therapy. The following is a session plan for such a group. The first step would be the Climate of Acceptance as will all remotivation therapy sessions. The second step, the Bridge to Reality, could take place as follows (the desired answer for each bounce question follows in parentheses):

1. What is the name for the surgery that each of you underwent? (total hip replacement surgery)
2. What are some precautions that one must follow after total hip replacement surgery? (cannot bend past ninety degrees)
3. What are some activities that may be more difficult for you since you cannot bend past ninety degrees? (bathing and dressing)

The therapist would then announce that the topic of the session is bathing and dressing after a total hip replacement surgery. In place of the poem, the therapist would show the group members the long-handled devices such as a dressing stick, a reacher, a sock aid, a long-handled shoehorn, elastic shoelaces, and a long-handled sponge. The therapist would then pass the objects around and allow the group members to look at them. After all of the objects have been passed around, the session would continue with step three, Sharing the World We Live In. During this step, the therapist would ask leading questions that would lead to a conversation on how one would safely use each of the devices. This could then be the transition into step four, An Appreciation of the Work of the World, when the group members themselves practice using the devices while the therapist assists them. After all of the group members have had an opportunity to practice using the devices, the therapist would begin the Climate of Appreciation by making a summary of the group session and then thanking each group member individually for coming.

The session that was just described is one example of how remotivation therapy can be used during the rehabilitation of self-care deficits. Remotivation therapy can also be adapted for use with many age groups and diagnostic groups.

Exercise Groups

Many professionals make use of physical exercises as part of their rehabilitation programs. Although exercise groups are common, exercise groups carried out through remotivation therapy are not. The following discussion illustrates how remotivation therapy can be used to conduct exercise groups.

Step one, Climate of Acceptance, is carried out in the same manner it would be during any remotivation therapy group. During the Bridge to Reality, the therapist would ask bounce questions that would establish the type of exercise that will be conducted during the session. Consider the following step two:

1. What is your favorite season of the year? (fall)
2. What type of sports are played in the fall? (football)
3. Name some of the positions on a football team? (kicker)
4. What body part does the kicker use during the football game? (legs)

At this point, the remotivation therapist or the group leader would announce that the group would focus on leg exercises. In place of the poem, the group leader could make use of exercise charts throughout the session. During step three, the leader could ask questions that would result in the group members giving instructions for exercises. For example, the group leader could ask, "What are some things that we do with our ankles?" This would lead group members to say things such as "tap our toes." The group members could then tap their toes ten times as an exercise.

After all of the exercises have been completed, step four would begin. During step four the conversation could focus on the benefits of exercise. The group members could discuss how exercise leads to decreased stiffness and increased range of motion, which assists with daily activities. The group could then discuss ways of doing exercise outside of the group to get exercise several times a day. After this discussion, the group leader would conduct the Climate of Appreciation.

Daily Living Skills Groups

The term daily living skills refers to the many activities that can make up a person's day. This includes activities such as cooking, cleaning, shopping, eating, etc. The rehabilitation of these skills often takes place in a group format and can be performed using remotivation therapy. The groups that were mentioned previously have made use of advanced remotivation therapy. Daily living skills groups, however, can be conducted through either basic or advanced remotivation therapy. The goal of the session determines whether basic or advanced remotivation therapy is appropriate. A cooking group that focuses on just baking a cake can be carried out through the use of basic remotivation therapy because the act of cooking is an objective topic. Teaching participants how to cook would be a subjective matter and, thus, would be advanced remotivation therapy.

The following session is based on a cooking group whose goal is to have group members bake a pie. Baking a pie is objective and, thus, is carried out through basic remotivation therapy.

No matter what skill a therapist is attempting to rehabilitate, the same format of remotivation therapy can be used. This includes conducting step one as usual. Step two would include bounce questions that would lead to the topic. A poem on the topic would then be read. Step three would consist of the group leader asking leading questions to provoke a discussion of the topic. Step four would be the actual activity. For example, if the remotivation therapy session is being utilized as a cooking group, step four would be the group members performing a cooking activity. The following is a complete remotivation therapy session that is being used as a cooking group:

Step I: Climate of Acceptance
Step II: Bridge to Reality
    1. What is your favorite meal? (dinner)
    2. What is your favorite course at dinner? (dessert)
    3. What is something that can be eaten for dessert? (pie)
    4. What are some types of fruits that are in pies? (cherries)
    The topic of our session is cherry pie.
Poem: "Cherry Pie" by Walter F. Pullinger Jr.
Step III: Sharing the World We Live In
    1. When was the last time you ate cherry pie?
    2. Where were you when you ate cherry pie?
    3. Who were you with when you ate cherry pie?
    4. What else do you eat with cherry pie?
    5. What can you put on your cherry pie?
    6. In addition to dessert, when can you eat cherry pie?
    7. Are there special times of year when you eat cherry pie?
    8. During which holiday meal(s) is cherry pie often eaten?
    9. What president is associated with cherries?
   10. Have you ever made cherry pie?
Step IV: An Appreciation of the Work of the World
    1. What kind of plate do you bake a pie in? (bring out pie tin after that response)

2. What ingredients do you need to make cherry pie? (ask this question until all ingredients have been mentioned)
3. What do you line the pie tin with?
4. What ingredients do you need to make pie crust? (ask this question until all ingredients have been mentioned)
5. What are the steps in making a cherry pie? (continue until pie has been completed)
6. What temperature should the oven be?
7. How long should the pie bake?
8. What utensils do we need to eat cherry pie?
9. Who can set the table?
10. What do we need to cut and then serve?

Step V: Climate of Appreciation

The session focused on making a cherry pie as an objective activity. The same session can be modified to teach participants the art of cooking to prepare them for independent living. For example, if the group members had all recently undergone a total hip replacement surgery and had to obey certain precautions (need to use a walker, not allowed to bend past ninety degrees, not allowed to twist the body, not allowed to cross legs, and not allowed to abduct knees), they may need to learn new functional mobility patterns to perform the act of cooking on their own. Since this type of session would involve the group members making a change in their lives, a subjective area, advanced remotivation therapy would be appropriate.

When conducting this type of session, the Climate of Acceptance would be conducted as usual. The Bridge to Reality and the poem would be the same as the session outlined previously. Step three, Sharing the World We Live In, would be a discussion of the functional mobility techniques that could be used in the kitchen so that hip precautions are followed. Step four, An Appreciation of the Work of the World, would then be conducting the activity while using the techniques learned in step three. The Climate of Appreciation would then be conducted in similar fashion.

The sessions just discussed show how remotivation therapy can be used to conduct cooking groups. The same format can be used to perform other activities such as making a bed, cleaning a room, etc. The questions need to be altered for different populations. Some of the questions in the first session may be too basic for older adults in a rehabilitation center but may be appropriate for long-term patients in mental hospitals.

Patient Education Groups

One of the important aspects of a rehabilitation program is educating patients about their diagnoses and their functional implications. This program is often best accomplished in a group since every group member is experiencing similar symptoms and similar functional deficits. The group members can also use one another as sources of support. Remotivation therapy, with its goals of increasing self-esteem and socialization, is optimal for conducting patient/family education groups.

When conducting patient/family education through remotivation therapy, the following structure is used. The Climate of Acceptance is conducted as usual. Step two would be slightly different since the group members will know in advance the topic of the session. Instead of asking bounce questions, the group leader could simply announce what the goal of the session is and ask the group members what they would like to learn during the session. In place of the poem, the group leader could make use of anatomical charts throughout the session. Step three would be a discussion of the condition itself and the functional implications of the condition. At this time a video that explains the condition may also be shown followed by a discussion of the video. Step four would be how the person can cope with these functional implications and continue to remain as independent as possible. The Climate of Appreciation would be used to conclude the session.

BASIC AND ADVANCED REMOTIVATION IN PSYCHOSOCIAL REHABILITATION

The groups that were discussed in the previous section were conducted using advanced remotivation therapy techniques with the exception of some of the daily living skills groups. The groups that will be discussed in this section, like the daily living skills groups, can be conducted using either basic or advanced remotivation therapy techniques. Each of the groups that will be discussed here can have multiple goals. The goals of the session will determine whether the group will use basic or advanced remotivation techniques.

Types of Psychosocial Remotivation Rehabilitation Groups

Media and Craft Groups

Media or craft groups are used in several programs for a variety of reasons. These groups, for example, can be used to teach group members leisure activities that they can perform. In this instance, the group could be conducted using basic remotivation therapy techniques since performing a leisure activity is something that each person can experience in the same manner. When the goal is to teach group members how to perform leisure activities, the basic remotivation therapy structure can be used.

The session would begin with the Climate of Acceptance followed by the Bridge to Reality. During the Bridge to Reality the group leader would ask bounce or nonlinear questions (Bierma, 1998) to establish the topic of the session (a craft or project in this instance). A poem that relates to the craft or project is then read to further develop the topic. Step three, Sharing the World We Live In, could be a discussion of how the craft or project relates to living. For example, if the project is a Christmas craft, the discussion in step three could be about Christmas in general and what crafts are associated with the holiday. Step four, An Appreciation of the Work of the World, is a discussion of the specific craft that is going to be presented and would include the materials needed to perform it and how it can be performed. This would be followed by the group members actually working with the craft or project. The session would end with the Climate of Appreciation.

Instrumental Activities of Daily Living (IADLs)

The term instrumental activity of daily living (IADL) refers to a higher level activity that a person typically performs during the day. Examples of IADLs include money management, homemaking, etc. Remotivation therapy can be used to facilitate the rehabilitation of these higher level skills. Since the rehabilitation of these skills will require a person to subjectively make a change in his or her life, the theories and structure of advanced remotivation therapy will be utilized with these groups.

The following is an example of how remotivation therapy can be used in the rehabilitation of the IADL of money management. The group leader would begin with the Climate of Acceptance to welcome group members. The following Bridge to Reality makes use of bounce questions, which establish the topic of the session:

1. What is your favorite meal during the day? (supper)
2. Where are some places that you can eat supper? (restaurants)
3. What do you need to take with you when you eat at a restaurant? (money)

At this point, a poem that is associated with money is read. The reading of the poem is followed by step three, Sharing the World We Live In. The discussion in step three would be a discussion of where and why money is used in restaurants. It would also include a discussion of the costs of certain items. Consider the following questions that would facilitate this discussion:

1. When you go to a restaurant, what tells you the cost of the items?
2. Are there restaurants that cost more than others?
3. What types of restaurants cost the most?
4. What types of restaurants cost the least?
5. After you are finished with a meal, what tells you the cost of the meal?
6. Where do you pay the check?
7. What are some things that you can do to decrease the cost of a meal?
8. Are there any other ways to spend money at a restaurant?
9. What are the standard percentages for leaving a tip?
10. What are some things that you can use to determine how much of a tip to leave?

Step three would be followed by step four, An Appreciation of the Work of the World. Step four could be a role-play about going to a restaurant. Some group members would be assigned the roles of waiter/waitress or customers while the remainder of the group members observe the role-play. The group member who is playing the role of the customer would be given a certain amount of money, a menu, and asked to order a meal. The member who is playing the waiter/ waitress would be given instructions to treat the customer in a certain manner. The customer would then be given a bill for the meal that he or she ordered. The person playing the role of the customer will be asked to pay the bill and to determine how much money to leave for a tip. After the role-play is completed, the observing group members would give the role-playing customer feedback on his or her performance.

The role-play would be repeated several times with different group members assuming different roles. Each time the role-play is repeated, different menus will be used. Some menus will be from expensive restaurants while other menus will be from less expensive restaurants. During each role-play, the role-playing waiter/waitress will be given different instructions on how to treat the customers. The goal of the session is to teach group members how to eat at a restaurant while living on a budget and how to determine what an appropriate tip is for service. The session would end with the Climate of Appreciation.

The session just described is one example of how remotivation therapy can be used in a money management group. The same format could be used during the rehabilitation of other IADLs.

Vocational Rehabilitation

Remotivation therapy can also be used as part of a vocational rehabilitation program. Similar to other groups that were discussed, vocational rehabilitation groups discuss subjective topics that require group members to subjectively make a change in their lives. Therefore, advanced remotivation will be utilized when remotivation therapy is used to conduct vocational rehabilitation groups.

The following is a description of one type of vocational rehabilitation group that can be conducted using remotivation therapy. The topic of the following session is how to set up a job interview and how to act during a job interview. The session would begin with the Climate of Acceptance. Consider the following Bridge to Reality, which establishes the topic of job interviewing:

1. What does one need to purchase items? (money)
2. What are some ways of getting money? (job)
3. When you want a job, what is the name for the initial meeting with the employer? (interview)

At this point, the group leader would announce that the topic of the session is job interviews. A poem that discusses job interviewing may be read at this point. Step three, Sharing the World We Live In, would include a discussion of looking for a job, setting up an interview, how to dress during an interview, and what to say and do during an interview. Consider the following questions that would facilitate this discussion:

1. Where is the first place you could look to find a job?
2. Which section of the newspaper lists jobs that are available?
3. After you find a job that interests you, what do you do?
4. When calling to request an interview, what are some things that you should say?
5. What do you do if you are not granted an interview?
6. If you are accepted for an interview, how should you dress?
7. What are some things that are inappropriate to wear during an interview?
8. When should you arrive at your interview?
9. What should you do and say when you first meet the person who is interviewing you?
10. What are some things that are appropriate to discuss during an interview?
11. What are some things that are inappropriate to discuss during an interview?
12. What should you do when the interviewer ends the interview?

Step three would be followed by An Appreciation of the Work of the World. This step would include group members watching videos of people who are taking part in job interviews. The group leader would ask group members to critique the job interviewee's performance. The group leader would then give feedback to the group members. The session would end with the Climate of Appreciation.

The session just described is one remotivation therapy session that can be used as part of a vocational rehabilitation program. Similar remotivation therapy sessions could be designed for other aspects of vocational rehabilitation such as writing a resume, etc.

CONCLUSION

This chapter has discussed how remotivation therapy can be used during both physical and psychosocial rehabilitation. Both basic and advanced remotivation therapy can be utilized to conduct rehabilitation groups depending on the goals of the group. With just a slight alteration in its structure, any rehabilitative process can be enhanced through the use of remotivation therapy.

REFERENCES

Bierma, J. (1998). *Remotivation group therapy: Handbook for the basic course.* York Harbor, ME: NRTO, Inc.

Gibson, A. (1967). *The remotivators' guide book.* Philadelphia, PA: F.A. Davis.

Meixsell, J. (1999). *Workbook of remotivation for the basic course.* York Harbor, ME: NRTO.

The New Merriam-Webster's Dictionary for Large Print Users (1989). Boston, MA: G.K. Hall & Co.

Robinson, A. (1967). *Remotivation technique.* Philadelphia, PA: Smith Kline & French.

Chapter 9

Conducting Remotivation in a Correctional Setting

James Siberski

This is the story of the author's nearly five years of experience working in a maximum security prison as a visiting remotivation therapist. Observations, even conclusions, contained in this story result from a systematic plan to investigate the common problems often associated with remotivation therapy: depression, isolation and alienation, poor motivation, apathy, and low self-esteem. Needless to say, the prison is fertile ground for developing and reinforcing behavior that keeps prisoners from seeing the outside world (or even their own inside worlds) as anything but negative.

Remotivation in this setting had many barriers to overcome, among them severe psychiatric disorders in the population: schizophrenia, depression, borderline personality disorder, and sociopathic personality disorder. Basic generic remotivation was included in the Pennsylvania correctional system but only as a *part* of an overall activity therapy program for inmates with psychiatric disorders. As reported elsewhere, inmates with psychiatric disorders are increasing at every level of correction and they are a difficult population to treat (Condelli, Dvoskin, and Holanchock, 1994).

This work was carried out with male inmates in a maximum security prison on a special needs unit. All had a psychiatric diagnosis. Their crimes ranged from robbery to drug dealing to homicide. They were referred to the program by prison counselors on the block to receive activity therapy. Once accepted into the program, the inmates received three hours of therapy a month, including remotivation therapy (Siberski, 2001).

This experiment proceeded for five years without the benefit of others' efforts. The literature contains scant information on which to plan a long-term program and make decisions about remotivation as used in a correctional setting and very little information is available on activity therapy. This extended program included an effort to obtain basic data about the effects of activity therapy, including both advanced and basic remotivation. Those results are reported in the *Journal of Offender Rehabilitation* (Siberski, 2001).

GOALS FOR ACTIVITY THERAPY

Four modest goals were established for this program that interrelated with inmates' issues and the overall correctional program goals:

1. The activity therapy program would prepare prisoners who had psychiatric and geriatric issues for a more advanced therapy.
2. The activity therapy program would support other ongoing therapy.
3. The activity therapy program would provide successful experiences for inmate participants.
4. The activity therapy program would develop old and new basic abilities of inmates.

As noted in the first goal, this experimental effort had the ultimate goal of increasing inmates' abilities to participate in higher therapeutic endeavors. In this sense, this effort provided more readiness preparation activities; in no sense did it intend to cure, treat, or address an inmates' diagnosis.

REMOTIVATION THERAPY

Remotivation therapy was selected because it fit into the activity therapy goals and limitations. In addition, remotivation therapy is sequential; that is, it can lead to a more advanced level of programming and therapy. Planning is provided by the guideposts used to conduct remotivation, and the five steps are the structure that the inmates require if they are going to advance in therapy. Inmates' participation was goal directed with each inmate having at least one long-term goal and one short-term goal.

When an inmate was admitted into the activity therapy program, each underwent an assessment, which included his activity interests, cognitive ability including verbal skills, and the presence of depression or depression-like features. Based on the assessments, the inmates were placed in remotivation therapy when they had not participated in groups prior to incarceration or when they showed a reluctance to participate in prison groups. The assessments also indicated that many inmates possessed low levels of educational achievement, for example, not finishing school. The inmates, in many cases, because they dropped out of school, denied themselves the opportunity to participate in groups and to socialize in their formative years. These social skill deficits made the inmate inappropriate for group psychotherapy (Metzner et al., 1998). This, however, is a deficit area that remotivation therapy can address. The assessment also indicated the preference for small groups, one-to-one interactions, or a preference to be left alone. This information was used to place inmates in either appropriately sized groups or one-to-one remotivation. The cognitive test, which was the mini-mental status exam, indicated sufficient verbal skills to participate in remotivation therapy.

The assessments showed that although inmates were functioning adults, they lacked group skills because of low levels of educational achievement. Their current psychiatric pathology was also provided. The assessments also showed skills that the inmates possessed in the past but which had atrophied because of the time they had spent in prison. If the inmate were to have a successful group experience, it would need to be structured, use objective materials, and work within the inmate's level or lack of expertise in groups. Furthermore, it would not appear to be therapy, since therapy implies "illness." Remotivation therapy seemed to meet those limitations for working with a correctional population.

Goals for Remotivation Therapy

Once the assessment is completed, the remotivation therapist must set reachable and realistic goals for the inmate. Having set reachable goals, the remotivation therapist must recognize that growth will be slow in this setting. Some examples of these goals are as follows:

1. The inmate will attend 50 percent of all scheduled groups to develop a pattern of participation and commitment.
2. The inmate will participate nonverbally in group as evidenced by looking at the speaker, making and maintaining eye contact, shaking hand of therapist upon entering and leaving room. This will begin to develop feelings of comfort in a group.
3. The inmate will answer one, two, or three direct questions in each remotivation session to begin to verbalize within a group.
4. The inmate will answer one nondirect question in each group to begin to develop more advanced group skills.
5. The inmate will spontaneously verbalize in a group to develop more advanced group skills.
6. The inmate will develop an appropriate behavior pattern, i.e., no verbal outbursts and no teasing or bullying in order to be able to participate in a group in a nonthreatening manner.
7. The inmate will make three small decisions in each remotivation session to begin to develop decision-making abilities.
8. The inmate will respond to one, two, or three other members in the group to begin to depend less on the therapist and participate more as a group member.

Planning for Remotivation Therapy

The following is a list of considerations that remotivation therapists should undertake before starting the program:

- *Payoffs for attending:* What is in it for the inmate? Some will get a payoff from the socialization; some will get a payoff from a good report that may affect their parole. Some will need a tangible payoff, which is the hardest to give in a prison setting. There are many restrictions that the remotivation therapist would not encounter in a "normal" community setting. Such social and physical elements as coffee, donuts, or cigarettes are not available within a prison setting. These payoffs will depend on the policies and procedures of the forensic institution for which you will be working. A certificate of accomplishment is a positive reinforcement for inmates, whether they are parole eligible or "lifers."

- *Location:* Having programs on the block will give you greater attendance than having programs in an outlying building. A gymnasium, library, or schoolhouse location would require the inmate to leave the block. If the inmate leaves the block, the prevailing weather condition becomes a factor affecting attendance. On-block activities will understandably have a greater attendance than off-block activities, especially when one considers the limited available payoffs. On-block groups will develop faster than off-block groups.
- *Degree of pathology:* The greater the degree of pathology, the more attendance in remotivation sessions will be affected. The inmates that will attend off-block activities are those with their pathology under greater control. The less depressed the individual, the better the attendance. Also, concrete activities are preferred over abstract activities.
- *Time:* It takes time for a program to develop. The inmates do not develop rapport quickly, and they do not trust. The climate of acceptance takes longer to develop in this population. The climate of acceptance is extremely important to develop no matter how long a time frame is required.
- *Education of staff:* When a remotivation therapist is starting out, he or she must define what remotivation therapy is and is not. What are the limitations and expectations as well as outcomes from remotivation therapy? These must be understood by the therapists, and communicated to the superintendent or warden, and especially to the guards. Prison staff may not understand why a remotivation therapist is sitting with eight patient inmates talking about cars in a remotivation therapy session. They will not know what to look for. It will look like a bull session when, in reality, the inmates are beginning to use very basic group skills, such as making small independent decisions in group, using old verbal skills, socializing adult to adult, and beginning to use cognitive skills such as remembering, imagining, and problem solving. Other planning considerations should be considered in the setting: type of inmate, philosophy of the prison or jail, and support of the administration that will need to be incorporated into the remotivation therapist's program.

DISCUSSION OF THE REMOTIVATION THERAPY APPROACH: THE FIVE REMOTIVATION STEPS

Step 1: The climate of acceptance in basic or advanced remotivation sessions.

Step 2: Therapists encourage participation, either nonverbally or, ideally, verbally and in a nondemanding way.

Step 3: A discussing, planning, and/or performing step.

Step 4: The action step of the session, involving some type of work or discussion of work.

Step 5: The traditional climate of appreciation.

The remotivation approach developed in this program never seemed to be threatening to our inmate group. All were quiet at first; later, inmates began to increase their member-to-member and member-to-therapist interactions as therapy continued. The climate of acceptance was rigidly adhered to, and inmates were reminded of this after each session. If they did not feel like talking, they did not need to. If they did not feel like staying, they would be excused. If they fell asleep, it was acceptable. Every inmate patient was always left with the expectation that their performance would improve in the future as they attended more and more sessions of remotivation therapy.

From the beginning, the therapist encountered very little negative behaviors from the inmate population. The behaviors that were noted included withdrawal behavior, one-/two-word answers, some teasing, and other behaviors that were considered nonsignificant. The important thing is that the groups were given an opportunity to develop skills at their own pace. When the climate of acceptance was used with the inmate population in the groups, attendance increased steadily. They learned to assimilate the remotivation structure gaining the understanding that there will be no surprises in store for them due to the adherence to the structure and that their behavior would be accepted within reason.

In Step 2, five to eight questions seemed to be the appropriate amount to lead up to the topic of the session. These questions needed to stimulate the inmates' interests and needed to be easy to answer. Questions about children were avoided because many inmates had committed child crimes. The therapist's participation in Step 2 was more active than in a nonprison group. The therapist may need to answer some of his or her own questions to get the group moving or to role-model the sought-after behavior.

Step 3 is conducted traditionally, for the most part. The therapist is at a disadvantage since the prison restricts the use of most audiovisual aids. Audiovisual aids were limited to magazines, pictures, and inmates' imaginations. The remotivation therapist must keep in mind that certain magazines and/or pictures might be restricted because of connections they would make to inmates' crimes.

Videotapes were used a great deal in the remotivation therapy sessions. These need to be cleared many days prior to the scheduled session. Sometimes this could cause a problem in the conduct of the remotivation group; however, the extra effort paid great dividends in therapy. Videotapes were quite useful in Step 3. After completing the Step 1 and 2 discussions, the inmates who were not used to participating in groups seemed to relish the break from verbal interaction that a short twenty- to thirty-minute videotape provided. The videotapes also provided an objective existence to the prison milieu for inmates. Tapes on animals provided much discussion about pets that the inmates had prior to entering prison. Videotapes on vacation cruises and places throughout the United States also were well received.

In a typical session, during Steps 1 and 2, leading up to the topic of "New York," a tape would be shown on New York that would replace the traditional poem. After the videotape, Step 3 would begin.

In Step 3, word search games and crossword puzzles were used. If the topic was "farm animals," a twenty-word crossword puzzle on farms would be used. The crossword puzzle questions were topic focused, and much discussion was held around the questions or the words in word search games. This provided a concrete activity in Step 3 for the inmates to engage in, which they seemed to enjoy.

Step 4 was, again, due to restrictions, a little difficult to conduct. Step 4 was generally limited to discussion, eliciting how one would change a tire, cook a roast, or plant a garden. The topic of jobs associated with cruise ships or newspapers was another common approach that was successful in Step 4 discussion.

Step 5 was the traditional climate of appreciation. Most inmates upon leaving offered to shake the remotivation therapist's hand to the point that inmates would wait in line. Simple thank-yous were used by the therapist while shaking the inmate's hand.

Remotivation was essential to the overall success of the activity therapy program in this prison setting. The remotivation structure was also used in other activity groups that the inmate experienced in the monthly meetings. Successful groups included mental health groups that educated the inmate about mental illness and groups that discussed personal values. This abstract topic would be considered in advanced remotivation. Inmates generally enjoyed the remotivation therapy program, believing that it was beneficial and that it prepared them for the future. There was an absence of disruptive behavior in groups; good attendance was observed, and inmates would suggest topics for upcoming groups (Siberski, 2001).

RECOMMENDATIONS AND CONCLUSION

The therapist should start with a group of about five to seven inmates and limit the group size to ten in any case. The time should not be more than an hour; less time is acceptable. A quiet, safe room should be available. Set the chairs in a circle prior to the inmates' arrival. Always have your session written out before the start of the group. Keep all topics basic and objective and omit subject matter that deals with children, sex, politics, legal issues, and religion. Allow six months for progress to occur. Inmates take longer to respond than other populations to remotivation therapy. The therapist will see that although the inmates will attend, they will remain quiet, superficial, and guarded for an initial period of time.

Basic and advanced remotivation therapy can be successful within the restrictive environment of a prison. It can meet the unique and varying needs of the inmate population and provide the therapist with a safe, structured program that moves inmates toward a more advanced level of therapy.

REFERENCES

Condelli, W., Dvoskin, J., and Holanchock, H. (1994). Intermediate care programs for inmates with psychiatric disorders. *Bulletin of the American Academy of Psychiatry and the Law* 22(1), 63-70.

Metzner, L., Cohen, F., Grossman, S., and Wettstein, M. (1998). Treatment in jails and prisons. In R. Wettstein (Ed.), *Treatment of Offenders with Mental Disorders* (pp. 211-264). New York: The Guilford Press.

Siberski, J. (2001). Response of psychiatrically impaired inmates to activity therapy. *Journal of Offender Rehabilitation* 33(3), 65-73.

Chapter 10

Use of Remotivation Therapy with Persons Who Have Huntington's Disease

Florinda R. Sullivan

Few people would disagree with the statement that self-esteem is critical to mental health. When a person's capabilities are restricted due to an illness such as Huntington's disease (HD), with little or no opportunity for self-expression, personal values may decline to such a degree that the will to live is lost. Improving self-esteem is critical to effective patient management.

An effective HD program permits the necessary flexibility in the range of services provided to carry out a creative attack by an interdisciplinary team knowledgeable about HD. This form of nondrug therapy, in partnership with appropriate medical management by a physician who understands the complexities of the treatment, will break down environmental barriers and expand the patient's opportunity for self-realization and fulfillment (Phillips, 1982).

OVERVIEW OF THE DISEASE

Although HD has been well researched and studied, most health care professionals have had little or no experience working with patients who have the disease. This lack of knowledge often leads to misdiagnosis and inappropriate treatment and placement of the HD patient in mental or correctional institutions.

HD is an inherited neurological disorder, named for Long Island physician George Huntington who first described it in 1872. It is a progressive disease that is always fatal. Damage to brain cells, especially to the caudate nucleus and the putamen in the basal ganglia, affects cognitive ability including thinking, judgment, movement, and emotional control.

Approximately 30,000 cases have been diagnosed in the United States, placing 150,000 people at risk of one day becoming HD patients. The autosonomal dominant gene that causes HD was identified in Boston in 1993. Each child of an affected parent has a 50 percent chance of developing HD, and a test has been developed for those at risk which can predict whether a person will develop HD. However, the test cannot determine when symptoms may appear. The average onset is between thirty and forty-five years of age. However, cases of onset have been documented as early as two and and as late as ninety. Personality changes may occur as early as ten years prior to diagnosis.

The average length of stay in a long-term chronic care facility for HD patients is five years at the end of life. In the advanced stages, 80 percent of patients are immobile; death usually occurs within fifteen to twenty years of diagnosis.

Symptoms and characteristics of HD can be divided into three areas of disorders: movement, cognitive, and psychiatric. These three categories of symptoms may vary through the different disease stages by individual and even by place in the family. To ensure successful management of the disease, therefore, a unique treatment plan must be developed for each person with HD.

Movement

HD affects both voluntary and involuntary movements. Involuntary movements are called chorea, an earlier definition of the disease. In the beginning stage, symptoms may include clumsiness, twitching, and lack of coordination. As the disease progresses, irregular movements such as jerking and writhing may occur and speech and swallowing are affected. In the more advanced state, the patient may become more rigid and lose all ability to swallow or communicate verbally. As mobility becomes more impaired and the likelihood of falls increases, a more protective environment is needed, including additional clutter-free space, padded walls and furniture, and specialized chairs and bedding.

The challenge for both patient and caregiver is to foster independence while balancing safety with freedom and risk taking. Although speech deteriorates in all patients, they may remain oriented and alert. The result of these aspects of the disease is often ineffective communication, frustration, and negative behavior. Ample time should be allowed for processing thought and verbalizing response. Verbal and visual cues should be offered as appropriate. For example, the patient might be asked to spell words or use aides such as an alphabet or communication board; conversations should be kept simple. Early consultation with a speech-language pathologist is important.

Eighty-five percent of patients experience difficulties with swallowing due to impaired voluntary control of mouth and tongue, impaired respiratory control, and cognitive changes. Weight loss is also a common problem for people with HD. Some evidence suggests that poor nutrition leads to increased movements, decreased swallowing and speech, and decreased alertness and responsiveness. A high caloric intake of 4,000 to 6,000 calories daily is recommended. Special attention to food texture, body position, and the need for adaptive equipment during feeding is essential for maintaining proper nutrition. Again, evaluation by a speech-language pathologist is recommended. Because of the ever-present danger of choking, patients with HD should not eat alone, and all caregivers should be trained in the Heimlich maneuver. Aspiration, pneumonia, and starvation are the leading causes of death.

Cognitive

The cognitive changes associated with HD are often more problematic than movement disorders. A decrease in executive function is evidenced by decreased ability for organization, sequencing, reasoning, planning, judgment, decision making, initiation, impulse control, emotional control, perception, awareness, concentration, memory, learning, language, and sense of timing. Memory is most affected by an inability to recall experiences that are stored in the brain. This affects both long- and short-term memory. The knowledge or concept may be intact, but the brain is unable to retrieve the information. Even minimal impairment in these functional abilities early in the disease can affect fulfillment of responsibilities at home or at work.

As the disease progresses, symptoms worsen, and tasks that were previously routine become a constant challenge. This can be overwhelming and lead to depression and loss of self-esteem.

Strategies for helping the patient cope with these changes include a calm and consistent environment, a structured daily routine, a written daily schedule, adequate preparation for changes in routine, attention to one task at a time, breaking the task down to simple steps, using verbal and visual cues, offering choices rather than using open-ended questions, and identifying and avoiding situations that trigger negative behavior.

When behavior problems occur, they are best managed by a non-coercive approach. Confrontation should be avoided. Rather than a punitive approach, gentle intervention and redirection can be most successful in averting crises.

Psychiatric

Psychiatric symptoms may occur before physical manifestations. This often leads to misdiagnosis and improper treatment, especially in the earlier stages of HD. Left untreated, the resulting changes in personality and behavior can cause diminished self-esteem, social isolation, divorce and/or family alienation, and loss of personal and financial success. The suicide rate can be as high as seven times the rate in the United States.

All HD patients experience personality changes and dementia as the disease progresses. Depression is the most common psychiatric problem. Other psychiatric disorders include bipolar disorder and obsessive-compulsive disorder. Additional symptoms include apathy, irritability, anxiety, delirium, disinhibition, sexual disorders, and schizophrenia-like disorders.

For the most part, psychiatric symptoms of HD are as treatable as they are in other patients. However, HD patients appear to experience more side effects of medications, especially those affecting speech, swallowing, and cognitive ability. When sudden changes in personality or behavior occur, the patient should first be evaluated for underlying physical or medical problems. For example, the patient simply may not be able to express that he or she is hungry, thirsty, cold, or in pain.

Social Implications

The average age of onset, the prime of life, and the genetic cause of the disease have serious psychosocial implications for both the patient and the family. Loss of social status, lost career opportunities, and financial stresses can be devastating. Experiencing the physical and mental degeneration of multiple family members can be despairing. The burden on "healthy" family members adds greater stress because they may be caring for more than one generation and even multiple siblings suffering from HD simultaneously. Often these same family members are involved in the care of young children of affected parents, who are also at risk. As noted previously, HD also imposes a significant financial strain. In 1977, the Commission for the Control of HD and Its Consequences computed figures of up to $234,000 for the direct lifetime cost of care for each patient.

REMOTIVATION: A PROGRAM MODEL FOR HD

Considering the available models to use to develop a program for HD patients at the Middlesex Hospital, Waltham, Massachusetts, remotivation therapy appeared to be the best choice. This was a specialty unit, internationally renowned for its clinical care of HD patients. The goal of Dr. Edward Bird, the director, was to provide optimal clinical care and to improve quality of life. The goals of remotivation therapy were most compatible with the need to address the psychosocial needs of the HD patients. Consequently, remotivation therapy would facilitate the dual objectives of Dr. Bird.

My first interaction with the HD patients was at the noontime meal. There I observed that two patients had thrown their trays. Two were removed to their rooms because of verbal abuse, and one patient was pacing and could not sit for the meal. The remaining patients were being fed or were self-feeding with great difficulty.

Mealtime has always been an important event in my household. As the mother of four, I always strived to have a pleasant meal in a calm environment, where we could share our daily experiences. What most overwhelmed me at this introduction to HD was the constant hubbub of that mealtime. The sounds of someone coughing or gagging were ongoing. At no time was the room still, as bodies were in constant choreic motion. I could not imagine feeding oneself while a leg, head, or arm was continually jerking. Their courageous attempts to help themselves instantly committed me to serving the HD community.

Although I knew remotivation would be the key to my program plan, I honestly did not know where to begin. Our course of study suggested the importance of a quiet environment free of interruptions. After observing the meal, that seemed unlikely. Offering juice as a stimulant was almost impossible because of swallowing difficulties. Some patients had gastric tubes. Others needed thickening agents, and others simply needed physical assistance. Serving juice could have used all the time allowed. Establishing criteria for joining the group was also a concern. Many patients who cannot speak and have a flat affect are often ignored. However, they may still be alert and oriented, and remotivation could be the tool to lead them from isolation. Sitting in the center on a rolling stool was not effective. Most of the HD specialty chairs are high off the ground and tilt back. Patients would be unable to see me if I was sitting on the stool.

Adjustments to Technique

The advanced course in remotivation therapy allows for more flexibility in the technique and would more nearly meet the objectives of the Middlesex HD program. Because of the identified problems, many adjustments were needed to accommodate the special needs of the HD patients. The location of the remotivation therapy session needed to be a space that allowed few interruptions by staff, loudspeakers, or other environmental distractions. Even with staff inservices, it was still important to make sure that before the group met, all patients were toileted and meds and other treatments administered. Large red stop signs were placed on doors to the room. Because so many patients were unable to communicate verbally, and because of the high level of absenteeism due to the lack of staff commitment to prepare members for group, the number of participants was expanded beyond eight. To compensate for not providing juice during the session, groups were held immediately after a high-caloric lunch. Patients were seated in a circle, and the therapist sat on a regular chair within the circle. This required an increased effort at maintaining eye contact and walking around the group with sensory aids.

Communication was probably the greatest obstacle to participation. Adjustments were made to the questions phrased using the five "W's" and "How" to accommodate nonverbal patients. An alphabet board was used for those who could point and spell a word. For those who could blink, questions were phrased for yes or no answers. The use of sensory aids was vital. They allowed group members to use their sense of smell, touch, hearing, and sight to appreciate more fully and comprehend the topic under discussion. Their responses to sensory stimulation allowed for improved assessment of participation in nonverbal patients and in patients with flat affect.

Often a patient would become disruptive. Procedure on the unit had been to remove the patient to his or her room which, in turn, caused further isolation. If all behavior is a form of communication, the professional must determine what the patient is trying to say. During remotivation therapy sessions, the strategy was changed to remove the person from the group, but to a quiet corner of the room.

Usually the group was interesting enough, especially if sensory aids were used to quickly recapture the disruptive patients' attention. Curiosity would often redirect their anger to the happenings of the group, and they would rejoin. Surprisingly, these episodes did not disrupt the rest of the group. Most participants, when given the opportunity, could express tolerance as many suffered these same uncontrollable outbursts.

Three series of twelve sessions were completed. Twenty individuals ranging in age from twenty-six to eighty-five participated, with an average age of fifty-four. Seven were male and thirteen were female. Length of stay varied from three weeks to nine years. Eleven were in specialty chairs, and seven were ambulatory. Twelve had moderate to severe dysarthria; of those twelve, eight were unable to speak at all. Five appeared totally unresponsive or withdrawn.

Initial topics chosen were very concrete and common to the environment and interests of all participants. All participants were given their own personalized folders to file poems, which they could later share with staff, family, or friends.

The group proved to be a positive experience from the start. All participants remained for the entire first session. The use of sensory aids proved invaluable as even the most withdrawn patients showed some response. Through the exploration of familiar topics, members became comfortable with participating. As interaction among group members was encouraged, patients began to more freely share their past experiences. They began to believe that their opinions and values mattered again. As one patient stated, "Everyone asks how are you, but no one stops to listen. Who really cares?"

In remotivation therapy, she learned that someone does care. With that knowledge, her ability to listen and concentrate improved. As group members became familiar with one another, greater respect and tolerance for each person improved. Personal self-esteem was reinforced because of a greater sense of self-worth; patients became more interested in their own rehabilitation goals. Many were able to return to their rehabilitation programs, previously abandoned because of noncompliance.

The group members began to build trust in themselves and those around them; they felt more comfortable in asserting their own needs. Their sense of belonging continued to grow with each session and absenteeism decreased. Prior to the implementation of remotivation therapy at Middlesex, behavioral outbursts of HD patients were problematic enough to have generated the formation of a performance improvement (PI) team. This team tracked the number of documented outbursts and the administration of PRN (as necessary) medications. The final report credited the dramatic drop in outbursts to the hiring of a remotivation therapist and to the presence of the medical director and the psychiatrist at weekly patient care conferences.

Program Expansion

The success of weekly remotivation sessions led to the overall expansion of programming from a few hours a week to six hours a day, five days a week. Advanced remotivation techniques allowed variety in the entire program. The interdisciplinary patient care team was used to support the program objectives as follows:

1. *Speech-language pathologist:* initial assessment and progressive evaluation of communication skills and dysphagia
2. *Nutritionist:* expertise for supplementary feedings to increase caloric intake
3. *Medical staff:* direction and evaluation
4. *Occupational therapist:* appropriate mechanisms to ensure participation and to encourage utilization in a social setting
5. *Physical therapist:* mobility assessment, development of a group exercise program
6. *Social service worker:* patient advocacy, family and caregiver involvement

All six hours of the program utilized the five steps of remotivation therapy. Specific goals and objectives were developed related to the restoration of self-worth, rekindling of social skills, real awareness, communication, and verbalization.

A typical day began with orientation, current events, and positive thinking. An exercise group was held three times weekly. Other groups included memory skills, reading, Bible study, movies, music, and dancing. A weekly basic remotivation group also continued. Special events were incorporated as appropriate.

For example, a basic session was held on homelessness two weeks before Thanksgiving. During the final summary, members decided to collect a food basket for a needy family from a church whose parishioners volunteered on the HD unit. Having little opportunity to purchase items themselves, patients traded favors with staff members. One patient promised not to throw her tray if staff donated two canned goods. She did not throw her tray for days, and the staff person donated a turkey in her name. This one session changed a time of great sadness for those hospitalized into a time of great self-satisfaction for what they could do for those less fortunate. One patient noted that at least he had food and a roof over his head.

The program was also used to problem solve for certain individuals. Sessions were held on personal hygiene and stealing when these issues became a concern on the unit. One-to-one sessions were also held for patients who were unable to attend regularly scheduled group sessions.

Outcomes of the Expanded Program

Outcomes were measured using the remotivation progress tool, the PI team tracking, and the rehabilitation team's chart of percentages of negative behaviors. All three tools showed positive results. The most significant scores on the remotivation progress tool were as follows:

1. A patient considered to be highly behavioral stayed in her room most of the day, ambulated only with maximal assistance; she was nonverbal and aggressive. Her initial score was 4. Her final score was 27. She began to speak, to walk with less assistance, and to participate in all program activities.

2. A patient with many daily outbursts went from an initial score of 20 to a maximum of 32, and had 0 outbursts during program.
3. Only one of twenty patients had a decrease in score. This patient expired before the end of the series.

The PI team report has been previously addressed. The rehabilitation team chart showed a decrease to 0 negative behaviors during program hours. There was no statistical measure of benefits to families and caregivers; however, through direct observation, I noted improved communication. Patients would proudly display their poetry books and generally were able to talk about their activities and new friends rather than their illness.

Families and staff were reminded that patients are real people with rich histories in a life prior to HD. They newly recognized these former teachers, engineers, homemakers, hairdressers, and electricians.

One gentleman who could only respond by blinking once for yes or twice for no was able to participate in group by some creative rephrasing of questions. Using Joyce Kilmer's poem "Trees" for the topic of autumn, we discovered that he had a definite aversion to raking leaves. The joy experienced by his wife when I asked her about his response was unbelievable. With tears in her eyes, she told us about all the maples on their property, and how John would start to complain every August about the inevitable task ahead. It meant so much to her that we had not only conversed with John but also had a few laughs.

Max Ehrmann's poem "Desiderata" was first published in 1948. This beautiful poem contains paragraphs that best capture the experiences of patients with Huntington's disease. One example is:

> You are a child of the universe,
> no less than the trees and the stars;

Several of my fellow remotivators have also used this poem in their sessions and as a key to understanding the heavy burdens of Huntington's disease and other degenerative diseases.

When asked about what topics she might like to see included in an education series on HD, one family member replied "Something positive. I'm so sick of hearing about disease progression and losses. Tell me, how do you live with HD?"

Remotivation is the instrument that helps to find the person behind Huntington's disease. When remotivation restores the person, the rewards are overwhelming to all: the person with HD, the family and friends, and the staff and caregivers.

The remotivation experience with HD patients echoes those words of Ehrmann, "in the midst of drudgery and broken dreams, it's still a beautiful world."

EPILOGUE

Over the past twenty-five years, I have developed a strong personal philosophy of nursing centered on a holistic approach to caregiving. Patients come to us with very individualized histories of life experiences. These histories make them the unique persons that they are today, and certainly affect their abilities to adjust to changes in lifestyle that illness may bring.

I have always had a keen interest in mental health, so I was very happy to receive information about a course in remotivation therapy. It seemed timely, as I had recently reentered the health care workforce after a ten-year sabbatical devoted to child rearing, community service, and assisting in the family business. Very early in the course I became excited about the possibilities of remotivation. It very quickly became a comfortable tool for me to use as I put my own personal philosophy into practice. My new position as program director for an agency providing day services to survivors of brain injury allowed me the opportunity to successfully integrate remotivation into the program schedule.

Upon leaving this position, I was employed by Middlesex Hospital as a remotivation therapist assigned to the Huntington's disease unit. Again, remotivation proved to be a successful tool for program design. However, in order to better understand how remotivation can be integrated into a program designed for an HD unit, the disease itself, its limiting aspects, and its implications for staff and caregivers must be studied.

RESOURCES

Huntington's Disease Society of America
158 West 29th Street, Seventh Floor
New York, NY 10001-5300

Phone: (212) 242-1968; 1 (800) 345-HDSA
Fax: (212) 239-3430
E-mail: <www.hdsa.org>

Huntington Society of Canada
151 Frederick Street, Suite 400
Kitchener, Ontario N2H 2M2
Canada
Phone: (519) 749-7063
Fax: (519) 749-8965
E-mail: info@hsc-ca.org
<www.hsc-ca.org>

For information on, or referral to, lay organizations in other countries, contact:

International Huntington Association
c/o Gerrit Dommerholt
International Development Office IHA
Callunahof 8
7217 St. Harfsen, Netherlands
Phone: 31-573-431595
Fax: 31-573-431719
E-mail: iha@huntington-assoc.com
<www.huntington-assoc.com>

BIBLIOGRAPHY

Ehrmann, Max (1927). Max Ehrmann's Desiderata from a wall poster by Athena International LTD, London, 1991.

Folstein, S.E. (1989). *Huntington's Disease: A Disorder of Families.* Baltimore: The Johns Hopkins University Press.

Myers, R. (1998). *Genetics and Testing for Huntington's Chorea.* Tewksbury Hospital Conference Presentation, Tewksbury, Massachusetts.

Paulsen, J.S. and Stoll-Fernandes, D. (1992). Understanding Behavioral Changes in Huntington's Disease: The Neuropsychology of HD and Strategies for Intervention. UCSD, Department of Psychiatry.

Phillips, D. (1982). *Living with Huntington's Disease.* Madison, WI: University of Wisconsin Press.

Rosenblatt, A., Ranen, N., Nance, M., and Paulsen, J. (1999). *A Physician's Guide to the Management of Huntington's Disease,* Second Edition. New York: Huntington's Disease Society of America.

Simpson, W. (1995). *Nursing Approaches for Clients with Huntington's Disease.* Horizons. Huntington's Disease Society of Canada.

Volicer, L., Hurley, A., and Mahoney, E. (1995). Management of behavioral symptoms of dementia. *Nursing Home Medicine* 3(12).

Wexler, A. (1995). *Mapping Fate: A Memoir of Family, Risk and Genetic Research.* New York: Random House.

Chapter 11

Remotivation Therapy in Nursing Care Facilities

Nancy Vandevender

Today, caregivers in various geriatric facility settings are faced with new challenges. These challenges call for new skills and a change in the approaches, delivery of service, and techniques currently in use. Increased demands on time, staffing, and the changing levels of residents' needs are challenging facility managers to re-evaluate the roles played by their various departments. Caregivers are charged with meeting the residents' needs while providing a quality-of-life setting. How can we achieve this goal? One of the many ways is by adding new skills and giving our staff the competency levels that are now required to fulfill the expectations of our residents. We need to adjust perceptions on the delivery of service to fit the residents' needs.

Many times we, as caregivers, try to make the residents fit into our programs and the facility's daily schedules. What we should be doing is adjusting our programs and daily schedules to fit the residents' needs and life experiences. How do we determine how to make these adjustments, and what are the factors involved?

Many factors may influence our decisions to choose programs and schedules for different residents. Today, the residents in our facilities vary from comatose residents, to those with cognitive and physical impairments, to those with dementia, to those needing minimal assistance, and to independent residents.

Each department is a component of the total facility, and all workers offer unique skills used in various areas to meet the needs of the residents. Each component is necessary as we strive to make our facility the best possible. At times we must readjust the facility programs and schedules to fit the residents' needs. Sometimes conventional programming and the daily routine does not work with everyone and adjustments need to be developed. Each resident is unique and requires adaptive approaches to aid in his or her adjustment period to a nursing home. Use of remotivation as a tool to facilitate this adjustment aids the staff as well as the residents and their families.

What are the benefits of using remotivation therapy in recreation activity and other areas of the facility? Considering the various levels of the residents, remotivation therapy can be used as a tool to fit programs for an individual's needs.

There are five levels of residents in long-term care settings; some settings have combinations of the levels. These levels include

1. Sensory: Those residents not able to participate in a group setting.
2. Cognitively and physically able to participate in a group: This group can also be subdivided into different levels of ability.
3. Cognitively and physically able but choose not to participate in a group: This group can also include some residents in a subacute setting.
4. Dementia: Those residents not based in reality at least 80 percent of the time.
5. Independent: Those residents with the ability to leave the facility unsupervised.

At each level remotivation therapy can be used as a tool to

- reach a nonresponsive or minimally responsive resident as a supportive tool,
- aid in the improvement/maintenance of cognitive/physical skills,
- assist the resident with resocialization skills,
- validate the resident's world of nonreality, and
- empower the resident toward independence.

To effectively meet the needs of each resident, workers in all disciplines need to be a part of the program that each resident acquires when he or she enters a facility.

Janssen and Giberson (1988) reported that a client group improved sensory abilities, group cohesiveness, and increased socialization.

The nursing department typically plays a larger role in facilities in relation to the other departments; however, all departments are needed
in order to make the facility programs function properly. Nurses, as
well as people in other departments, can use the five-step technique:

- Nurses use it when they need to assist the residents with baths,
  medications, and ADLs.
- Social service workers use it as a bridge when new residents are
  admitted and find the process long and confusing.
- Housekeeping/maintenance employees use it when cleaning or
  repairing the residents' rooms.
- Dietary workers use it to address food needs of residents by facilitating groups to assist with menus and food service.
- Employees in rehabilitation departments (occupational therapy
  [OT], physical therapy [PT], speech therapy) use it in conjunction with their specialized therapy programs.

People from each discipline can be trained to effectively use
remotivation within their own specialty areas to serve the residents'
needs. Remotivation therapy has been the best kept secret in the facility by the recreation activities department. One purpose of the recreation activities department and the goals of remotivation are the
same, to be a "nonthreatening" therapy. Our efforts seek to create a
supportive environment in which the resident can achieve goals and a
quality of life that uses past leisure experience and work skills.

So, just how can remotivation therapy help us to achieve our quality-
of-life goals? Now is the time to let the secret out. Remotivation therapy can be used by every staff member in long-term care facilities. By
learning this alternative approach, remotivation therapy can be used
easily, as a one-to-one intervention or in a group setting, by people
from every department in the facility. Using remotivation can make
all the difference when attempting to create recreation programs and
a pleasant environment to enhance the quality of life that meets the
residents' needs. Care plan development can be enhanced by adding
remotivation therapy goals and approaches.

Remotivation therapy can be easily adapted to several interventions. It can be used in a one-to-one intervention. At times residents
can socially isolate themselves or perhaps they are so impaired that a
group setting is inappropriate. In this scenario it may be best to ap-

proach the individual in his or her room or in a quiet setting. A five- to ten-minute remotivation session may contain all the information the resident can assimilate at one time.

The optimal setting is when remotivation therapy is used in a group session. During a group, the facilitator motivates the various cognitive, physical, and social skills of the residents who are involved. The typical remotivation group has eight to twelve residents. Remotivation can be used in a large or small group with appropriate planning and organization. As a staffing bonus skill, it can be adapted to presentations often made during orientation or yearly facility mandated inservice training.

How can we be sure the remotivation session is correct or "a proper fit" to meet the residents' needs? The development of a session can be done only with appropriate information and training. The five steps in the remotivation session are key to success. Planning and resource management are the tools that are used to make sure the remotivation therapy session fits properly. Background work and organization is essential to all sessions. A hastily put together program or one-to-one intervention will not have the same positive results as a well-defined and assembled group session or intervention.

Due to the unpredictability of the residents' involvement, the facilitator needs to be flexible in approaching the topic and even in choosing the topic itself. Resource material can be obtained from many sources (see Box 11.1). Residents, family, and other staff/team members can be valuable resources and should be called upon. These are

---

BOX 11.1. Additional Resources for Session Topics

- Chase's Calendar of Events
  NTC/Comtemporary Publishing Group, Inc.
  4255 W. Touhy Ave.
  Lincolnwood, Illinois 60712-1975
- *Ideals* magazines (check yard sales and card stores)
- The Mimi Page (in many newspapers)
- Residents' families
- Staff members in the facility (hobbies, singing groups)
- Residents: check their assessment sheets for work and leisure history
- Seasonal themes
- Local history, attractions

the tools that workers from each discipline can use to integrate remotivation therapy into their area of expertise. The trained therapist can be a valuable consultant to each discipline in the development of interventions to be used.

The use of remotivation should not be limited to the recreation activities department. Pennsylvania State University has published a manual of human relations that deals with the training of staff to "promote sensitivity, empathy and skill in working effectively with the older individual" (Fleishman, 1976, p. 97). The manual is divided into several sections, with the third section devoted to establishing a nursing home remotivation program. Employees in all other departments could and should be trained to use remotivation therapy to enhance their unique skills and perspectives. For instance, workers in the dietary department could use it to incorporate residents into the planning of meals and even into some stages of meal preparation. Gardens can be established that would promote staff and resident interaction as well as a sense of accomplishment and pride. Research into the cultural needs of a diverse population can lead to better understanding of the nutritional and cultural backgrounds of the residents.

Nurses can use remotivation therapy techniques to enable staff to be more responsive and empathetic. The nursing staff can spend quality time reminiscing about the past and learning about their residents. Using preplanned one-to-one sessions, nurses can begin to build the trust relationship between themselves and the residents.

Employees in the social services department need to work closely with the recreation activities department as both departments take detailed accounts of the residents' histories. This information is used in the development of goals and in problem resolution. Many residents face issues when leaving their homes and moving into long-term care facilities. The social service department is charged with helping residents to cope with these lifestyle changes.

The housekeeping/maintenance personnel can benefit from remotivation training by using the technique when cleaning or repairing items in the residents' rooms. It could heighten the employees' awareness of changes in the residents' status and they could then report these observations to the appropriate department. It would also give these staff members more of a relationship to the residents than is typically found in nursing facilities.

A group of people not directly involved in resident care, but more with family interactions, includes not only the administrator and director of nursing, but those in the ancillary services of accounting, personnel, medical records, and staff development.

Remotivation techniques can be applied to new staffing orientation and to assist families in the transition from home to facility life. Proper training is essential for new staff to grasp the therapeutic use of remotivation therapy.

The development of remotivation therapy skills will come through training and implementation of these techniques. Creating the remotivation session may require trials and adaptations. You do not often go into a shoe store and buy the first pair of shoes you see. So it is with remotivation: Learning how, when, why, where, and what are the first steps toward creating effective sessions and techniques. Session topics can be developed by using the resident assessment sheets, conversations with families, seasonal themes, and using many resources (see Box 11.1 for examples).

Props are an essential ingredient in the remotivation session. They serve as a visual tool to draw the resident into a verbal exchange. As a visual stimulant to bridge the resident from the past to the present, props are invaluable. The props need to be large enough to handle, especially when working with a lower functioning group that needs the additional sensory component.

Development of the five steps of a session can be almost as enjoyable as doing the session. Each step can be used by a variety of departments during their daily interactions with a resident/patient. The following is an example of how nursing staff could use remotivation in their daily contact with a resident.

1. *Climate of acceptance:* Designed to make the resident feel worthwhile and welcome and to enhance interaction. This is accomplished by a handshake, a friendly greeting, or a compliment; or calling the person by name and introducing yourself, even if you believe that the person would know you. Each employee should take this approach whenever and wherever he or she meets a resident. "Hello, Mrs. Smith. You look very nice this morning. My name is Nancy and I will be your aide today."

2. *Bridge to the real world:* Designed to bring the resident to understand what it is that you are about to do, e.g., give a bath. The

staff might sit with the resident and begin to talk about a general topic such as flowers and develop the topic so the end concept is a bath. For example, "Mrs. Smith, did you ever have a flower garden? What do you need to raise beautiful flowers? What happens to the dirt when it gets rained on? Did you ever play in the mud when you were a little girl? What did your mother do? Well, that's what we are going to do now: take a bath."

3. *Appreciation for the work of the world:* Designed to bring the residents to as much reality as they feel is comfortable. During this step the staff person will explain the bath set-up (as it will be very different from the ones in the resident's past). For example, "Mrs. Smith, what should we do first now that we are in the tub room? How should you get into the tub? Here, let me show you how." (If the resident needs assistance to bathe, ask if you can help. If not, retreat slowly and let the resident do as much as possible for himself or herself, praising the resident's independence).

4. *Sharing the world we live in:* Designed to have the residents relate their experiences with the topic. The staff person will, at this point, ask the resident what would be needed to take a bath. As the resident relates items, the staff person begins to gather them and place them with the resident. Also, at this time, the staff person can begin to take the resident to the tub room while engaging in conversation. This will relax the resident. He or she will become part of the process, thereby eliminating stress and possible combativeness. When approaching the tub room begin to relate how the bath has changed and ask for the resident's remembrances.

5. *Climate of appreciation:* Designed to bring closure to the session or interaction. This step gives validation to the residents for their participation. For example, "Mrs. Smith, I would like to thank you for letting me help you with your bath. I have enjoyed talking to you today. May I come in again to see you?"

Training the entire staff in the techniques of remotivation therapy will complement all the other tools and procedures already in existence to make your facility a warm, safe, and comfortable place for your residents. Using remotivation techniques will effectively help your staff to achieve the ultimate goal: enhancing the quality of life for the residents/patients and clients placed into your care.

BIBLIOGRAPHY

Aday, Ronald H. and Aday, Kathryn L. *Group Work with the Elderly: An Annotated Bibliography.* Westport, CT: Greenwood Press, 1997.

Banik, Sambhu N. and Tierney, Gail M. "Tri-Dimensional Approaches in Working with a Geriatric Population in a Chronic Disease Institution." *Nursing Homes,* September-October 1982, 31(5), 17-19.

Brennan, Jim. *Memories, Dreams and Thoughts: A Guide to Mental Stimulation.* American Health Care Association, Washington, DC, 1981, p. 191.

Capuzzi, Dave, and Gross, Doug, and Friel, Susan E. "Recent Trends in Group Work with Elders." *Generations,* Winter 1990, 14(1), 43-48.

Day, R.R. "Integrative Group Approach for Treating Dysfunctional Elderly." *Nursing Homes,* September-October 1981, 30(5), 38-40.

Fleishman, J.J. *Manual of Human Relations for People Working with the Elderly: Theory and Practice.* Pennsylvania State University, 1976, p. 97.

Forsythe, Emma. "One to One Theraputic Recreation Activities for the Bed and/or Room Bound." *Activities, Adaptation and Aging,* 13(1-2), 1988; 1989, 63-76.

Hern, Brenda G. and Weis, David M. "A Group Counseling Experience with the Very Old." *Journal for Specialist in Group Work,* September 1991, 16(3), 143-151.

Holmes, Elizabeth A. and Everline, Diane. "Use of Volunteers in Social Group Work as Remotivation Leaders." *Journal of Long Term Care Administration,* Winter 1984, 12(4), 9-12.

Janssen, Judy A. and Giberson, Dawn L. "Remotivation Therapy." *Journal of Gerontological Nursing,* June 1988, 14(6), 31-34.

Koh, K., Ray, R., Lee, J., Nair, A., and Ho, T. "Dementia in Elderly Patients: Can the 3R Mental Stimulation Program Improve Mental Status?" *Age and Aging,* May 1994, 23(3), 195-199.

Maloney, Charlotte C. and Daily, Terran. "An Eclectic Group Program for Nursing Home Residents with Dementia." *Physical and Occupational Therapy in Geriatrics,* Spring 1986, 4(3), 55-80.

Murphy, Mary C., Conley, Jane, and Hernandez, Margaret. "Group Remotivation Therapy for the 90's." *Perspectives in Psychiatric Care,* July-September 1994, 30(3), 9-12.

Needler, Willa and Baer, Mary Ann. "Movement, Music and Remotivation with the Regressed Elderly." *Journal of Gerontological Nursing,* September 1982, 8(9), 503-697.

Sulman, Joanne and Wilkinson, Sue. "Activity Group for Long-Stay Elderly Patients in an Acute Care Hospital: Program Evaluation." *Canadian Journal on Aging,* Spring 1989, 8(1), 34-50.

Zgola, Jitka M. and Coulter, Linda G. "I Can Tell You About That: Therapeutic Group Program for Cognitively Impaired Persons." *American Journal of Alzheimer's Care and Related Disorders and Research,* July-August 1988, 3(4), 17-22.

Chapter 12

Elements of Style and Techniques in a Mental Health Hospital

Frances Kay Vickery
John J. Allison

If the essential core of the person is denied or suppressed, he gets sick sometimes in obvious ways, sometimes in subtle ways, sometimes immediately, sometimes later.

Abraham Maslow

THE GROUP FORMATION PROCESS

Soon after our introduction to remotivation therapy, we surveyed our wards and found a group on the geriatric psychiatric men's ward who were not participating in regularly scheduled programs. We found a group who did not meet the qualifications for other forms of treatment offered, except containment on a locked ward and psychiatric medications. The treatment team agreed that we could provide a remotivation group program. Also, we agreed that the individuals we had selected were in need of more interpersonal forms of treatment than they were currently afforded.

We scheduled a time and place for the group and began to organize sessions. We met to consider the particular needs of our select group members and consider topics for our first program. Of course we started with basic remotivation. The men we had selected would, at best, respond to the basic model.

Having an all-male group was an asset because we could focus on topics of interest to most men, such as cars, work, trucks, and job skills.

Later we focused on topics on the women's ward such as cooking, gardening, and topics of interest to most women. We also had a series of groups on "spiritual empowerment in the treatment mall."

We began the climate of acceptance on an individual basis. We would go on the ward, attempt to find our people, and decide on the spur of the moment who would find which person. Each person was led to the room individually allowing time for conversation to begin as soon as we approached a patient. Some were in wheelchairs and some were in gerichairs. We talked with them as we moved them from the dayroom to the meeting room. We then acknowledged each person by name and thanked him or her for coming to the group. Any social problem that came up at the beginning would be resolved immediately. We rearranged seating according to need. Of the seven men we selected for the men's group, two failed to participate as expected and were discontinued. Now and then we had to retrieve persons who started group and then left for the rest room and did not find their way back.

THE SESSIONS

Some Topics from Our Remotivation Sessions

Some of the basic remotivation topics we used in our group sessions were

- what I did for a living,
- memories of early school years, and
- my home when I was a child.

From the responses these men gave us, we thought we had a good chance to succeed with advanced remotivation topics.

Some of the advanced topics we used were

- attention: that is to say, being alert, discovering the world around us;
- being present in the moment, the time line of life;
- compassion: the necessity to care and be cared for;
- forgiveness: feeling the healing balm of being forgiven;

- hospitality: allowing people into your heart;
- joy: the right to be happy in life; and
- justice: what is fair.

We also touched on other topics such as oppression and equality.

Debriefing

One thing we learned from debriefing was to build one session on another according to our group's responses. This offered relevance to each session while keeping it fresh with new concepts and keeping good continuity of care. In addition, we were careful to connect this organization of sessions to good documentation, including the short-term and long-term goals of the patient.

In these debriefing sessions the following also need to be answered:

- Was the remotivation form properly used?
- Were the short-term goals of the patient met?
- Were the treatment team's goals for the patient met?

All of these questions led to good documentation.

The Importance of a Cotherapist

We learned the importance of working not alone, but with a cotherapist. The second person can observe the reactions of the group members and the presentation of the material—a good observance of the material is extremely important for the writing and execution of further sessions. The coleader is also valuable for the evaluation of the presenter, of what he or she is and is not saying. Another value of the coleader is to note the social and psychological reactions of the group members. A practical asset for a coleader is that two leaders are safer than one. Most important when a session is over, both the presenter and coleader conduct the debriefing session.

CASE STUDIES OF OUR GROUP MEMBERS

Although the therapy was successful with all five of the men's group participants, we present two case studies only. The purpose of the case studies is to demonstrate that basic and advanced remotivation groups are effective for even "backward," treatment-resistant patients.

Charlie

Charlie was a seventy-two-year-old man who had severe bipolar disorder and cycled about twice a month. At his age, the manic stages were fairly well controlled to prevent him from falling or instigating arguments with his peers, but the depressed stages were seemingly impenetrable. He could not even blink his eyes to acknowledge when he was being spoken to. His treatment goals were

- to decrease anger and fights with peers,
- to decrease the incidence of falling and sustaining injuries, and
- to improve stability of mood.

Charlie, now deceased, suffered from chronic type bipolar disorder, which was partially controlled by medications. Nevertheless, he benefited from remotivation therapy. At times, Charlie was not able to say one word throughout the entire session because he was severely depressed. During these periods he was virtually immobile, yet during his manic phases we realized how much he really did comprehend during his "down" phases. During the manic phases he explained to us that he was quite able to listen to and remember everything that happened during his depressive periods.

As part of an ongoing group for a year and a half, Charlie had the support of the members of the group in the following ways: Freddie, who is severely withdrawn and depressed, gave his support and friendship via prayer and compassion. George, who is schizophrenic, demented, and who can hardly see, helped ease Charlie's emotional distress through words and deeds of kindness. Richard, who was brain damaged and antisocial, would push Charlie's wheelchair up to the table for him during meals, put his napkin on him, and get things for him during a meal. This type of compassion came about as a result of the exchange of ideas developed in the group. Remotivation therapy opened up the avenues that enabled the participants to demonstrate compassion, care, and companionship in all of these men's lives. The group worked. The men in this group were able to take the concepts and understandings developed in our remotivation sessions and apply them in many aspects of their lives. Charlie, as a member of this group, functioning with it even during his periods of deep depression, enjoyed living among friends and was able to die with dignity. At his funeral, Deacon Allison had the privilege of performing his eulogy and mass sermon as a guest of the Russian Orthodox Church. Remotivation therapy opened doors for us that we had imagined to be permanently closed.

Freddie

Freddie is a seventy-nine-year-old male Mennonite farmer who suffers from severe depression and dementia. He spent years alone in a trailer shunned by family and friends. In that trailer, which was in the middle of an abandoned field, he lived in poverty. He had no running water or toilet facilities. He had little heat and very little food. After many years living in such a pitiful state, his family put him in our hospital. Upon arrival with us he was very withdrawn, very depressed, and physically ill. We knew from the family that he was divorced from his wife and that he was not allowed to see her or his two daughters by court order.

Freddie, as a rule, stayed in bed complaining that he was in "snake country." When he was out of bed, he groped females and made lewd suggestions to them. Later on he identified himself to the team and others as a five-star general in the air force. He even recruited his peers into the air force. His treatment goals were

- to cease inappropriate sexual approaches to women,
- to decrease delusional ideation (that he was a general), and
- to be less withdrawn and more able to socialize in order to participate in skill-building therapeutic activities and to improve social and vocational skills.

When we selected Freddie to participate in our group he could not really express his physical or mental pain. He just kept using the same expressions over and over:

"Is it time for a cigarette?"
"I'm a five-star air force general."
"I'm a pilot, you know."
"I'm in snake country."
"I'm rich."

It took many sessions in group before he could speak on the topics we were discussing. For instance, Freddie told us about his little dog Bobby dying when he was a child. This was his first real communication. He told us about his home and his school, especially the teacher he had from first through eighth grade. He told us about being a pilot and owning his own airfield and his own plane. He told us about being in snake country, which I knew meant that he thought he was sick and going to die. He revealed to us that he was a conscientious objector. He stated that he signed up for two years working as an operating room technician at the army air force base at Denver, Colorado. There he was ridiculed and belittled for being a conscientious objector and living up to his faith.

After more group sessions, Freddie communicated to us that he was shunned by his family. He told us about his mother and father and his wife and children, but in fragments and with deep regret. He revealed that he was divorced and could not see his ex-wife and his two daughters. Freddie also thought he was shunned by his church.

RESULTS OF OUR MEN'S GROUP

Although the actual text in a remotivation group might be about "your best friend when you were a kid," the cumulative effect is improvement of self-concept, self-esteem, and social skills. This leads to less need to communicate through aggression and threats, less dependence on peculiar ideas to support self-concept, less attention seeking, less demanding behavior, and more self-reliance and ability to negotiate one's way through life with less stress and less flight into psychosis.

As you can see from the positive aspects of this group, remotivation group therapy does promote participation and companionship and reinforce friendships and companionships. It does bring about change. It does increase self-esteem. It does promote social skills and increase interaction among the group members and others outside the group. And it certainly does increase a spirit of hope and courage for its members. As you can understand from what has been discussed, it can change "takers" into caregivers. It offers support to other groups, fellow patients, staff, and family members. Most of all, what we have done with this group demonstrates the positive aspects of remotivation group therapy. It was the epitome of the use of "remo" to develop and bring out the positive aspects of each participant for his benefit, and for the benefit of the ward milieu.

During the advanced remotivation groups we used a Celtic poem as our audiovisual. The men loved it. The most amazing result is that they created a beautiful Celtic poem using the style of our audiovisual. Their poem is indeed a Celtic poem based on ancient "oral tradition," a tradition that is one of the oldest of humankind. In this oral tradition the one who is speaking becomes one of the elements of nature and in that personification makes things occur that are natural and everyday, thus, giving pleasure to the listener. Each man in our group voiced part of the poem that appears here. Remember this poem was voiced in the Celtic oral tradition by men not even allowed off the ward to eat and who cannot read or write because of their mental illnesses.

Think about the real meaning of the words as well as the love, hurt, consideration, and healing thoughts they convey.

The Wind's Monologue

I am the wind. I am soft and gentle. I am swift and terrible. I go where I like. You can feel me but you cannot grab me, for I am the wind.

I gently blow over the wheat field making it look like the sea, making each head bow down to its maker.

I sometimes blow across little daisies making them do their ballet. And, oh yes, I pick up beautiful scents of all the flowers and grasses after a rainstorm and gently stir them for people to enjoy.

I can flip your favorite hat off your head. I can cool you on a hot day. I can gently blow across an old woman's veil moving it aside so I can kiss her cheek, for I am the wind.

But I have my moods. At times I am terrible in my anger. I twirl myself into tornadoes. I rip up great oak trees. I toss them into the air and smash them on the ground like matchsticks, for I am the wind.

I blow mightily over the sea picking up moisture, making the waves mountains, and then I smash them against the shore—destroying docks, sinking ships, ruining beaches, blowing cars and trucks off the road.

Then I slow down, slowly rain and wash your cars, your roofs, your roads, and you. I blow the rain wherever I want. I make it go in different directions.

Then I stop and blow everything dry, for I am the wind.

I love to push against the clouds making them form all kinds of beautiful shapes. I can make them drift or send them flying, for I am the wind.

I blow the winter rain across roads and make ice. I freeze lakes to give people fun. I blow around those people and I make them fall. I playfully make fools of them, for I am the wind.

I am the wind and I love you.

Chapter 13

Remotivation and Alzheimer's Disease

James Siberski.

INTRODUCTION

Alzheimer's disease is the most common cause of dementia. During the course of this disease multiple cognitive deficits occur, including memory impairment, language disturbances, an inability to carry out motor activities, failure to recognize objects, and disturbances in planning, organizing, and other executive functions. It causes significant impairment in social and occupational functioning and is characterized by gradual onset and continuing cognitive decline (American Psychiatric Association, 2000). Alzheimer's disease affects two groups of people: those with the disease and the loved ones who care for them (Medina, 2000). Although remotivation therapy can benefit both groups, this discussion will focus on the individual with the disease.

Since remotivation therapy is a therapy that works with an individual's strengths and unwounded areas, it is well suited for those affected by Alzheimer's. Although little literature focuses on it, many cognitive and social abilities apparently remain unaffected by the progression of the disease (Sabat and Collins, 1999).

The goal of treatment is to prevent excess disability. Excess disability is defined as the discrepancy that exists when a person's functional incapacity is greater than that warranted by the actual impairment (Sabat and Collins, 1999). In other words, their functional loss is caused by disuse or atrophy rather than disease.

BENEFITS FOR ALZHEIMER'S PATIENTS

Remotivation therapy can tap into a host of cognitive functions ranging from initiation of social contact, affectional warmth, manifestations of selfhood, humor, and helpfulness to mention a few cognitive functions. Remotivation is enhanced by the availability of medications that target the symptoms of Alzheimer's disease as well as medications that will control some of the behavioral manifestations of the disease. The result of utilizing the intact cognitive functions and utilizing the appropriate medications makes possible a slowing of the progression of the disease by preventing atrophy and maximizing use of the unaffected areas of the brain.

Clients greeting other clients, shaking other clients' hands, and spontaneously talking to others in the group can be seen as initiation of social contact in remotivation therapy groups. Affectional warmth can be seen when clients reach out and shake hands, smile at other group members, and laugh in group. Manifestations of selfhood are seen when clients respond to questions with "I," "me," "mine," and "my," indicating the client's point of view. An example of this in remotivation therapy would be the response to the question "What's your favorite color?" or "Where is your favorite place to visit?" to mention two examples. Clients also are helpful to one another by assisting other clients in finding words, remembering details, and offering suggestions. These are but a few areas where remotivation can focus on the intact abilities of a client with Alzheimer's disease. Remotivation can also prevent these functions from developing excess disability or atrophy.

Remotivation therapy can meet the following objectives required to provide meaningful activity therapy to this client group. The objectives are

- to focus on abilities and not weaknesses,
- to provide a purposeful use of time and a sense of cohesiveness,
- to support desired behaviors, and
- to foster communications on both the verbal and nonverbal levels (Hellen, 1998).

Remotivation therapy targets the client's strengths and avoids weak and wounded areas thereby focusing on the positive abilities of clients. It fosters group cohesiveness by structuring the group in a circle. It is a purposeful use of time since it would be normal to find a group of older individuals engaged in conversation at most times of the day. It is desired behavior with clients who have Alzheimer's disease to maintain their abilities to socialize, maintain attention, and share their memories and to challenge those abilities that have been retained.

Finally, remotivation can support the client's abilities to communicate through its questioning technique. Clients are asked simple questions—bounce questions, easy-to-answer questions, clue-giving questions—that enable them to verbally respond on an adult level. Those who cannot respond on a verbal level can be engaged through the use of visual aids. The therapist can present a picture of a cluttered basement asking the client to point to an object that he or she recognizes. The therapist then can verbally identify the item that the client chose, identifying it, and telling about the item. This allows the clients with Alzheimer's disease to nonverbally participate in remotivation therapy.

The previous discussion briefly outlines how remotivation therapy can successfully meet the criteria for providing meaningful activity to the Alzheimer's client. With practice the remotivation therapist can improvise on the verbal or nonverbal interactions of the client. The technique relies on the experience of the therapist in the use of the questioning technique.

THE PROCESS

Patient Evaluation

The remotivation therapist, in an effort to provide meaningful activities to the clients, must evaluate each client on four levels. The first level requires the therapist to determine what physical abilities are required and what physical abilities the client has retained. These include but are not limited to dexterity, speed, and coordination. The remotivation sessions must be adapted to any limitations that are present.

Sensory abilities would then be evaluated including, but not limited to sight, hearing, and smell. If the therapist planned on a step four where clients would bake a cake, sight and smell would be two sensory abilities the therapist should assess, since measuring ingredients would require sight, and appreciating the aroma of the cake would require smell.

The third area to be assessed would be perceptual abilities, including but not limited to eye-hand coordination and spatial relationships. Last, cognitive functions that are still intact should be assessed, including but not limited to communication, problem solving, attention, and judgment (Handy, et al., 1994).

If the therapist, in planning a remotivation session, does a competent evaluation, the outcome will be successful. It will avoid failure. This would give the patient a sense of accomplishment and provide meaningful normalizing social interaction.

The Sessions

Remotivation should be scheduled once or twice a week in the same location with the same therapist and should be limited to approximately thirty-five minutes. The number of clients in a group will usually be five to seven; however, the degree of impairment may dictate as few as four or five. The environment should not be over stimulating because it will distract the client. The therapist should ensure that the client's sensory deficits are addressed in a positive manner. This means they should have their glasses on and hearing aids in and working; they should be dressed appropriately for an adult. If the therapist is utilizing audiovisual aids, they should be large enough to accommodate for age-related changes in touch, taste, smell, hearing, and vision.

The remotivation therapist will need to listen closely and be very involved in the group's responses to the therapist's questions. Depending on the clients' levels of cognitive impairment, they may answer the questions in a rambling, circumstantial, or tangential manner requiring the therapist to restate the answer so that it is more understandable to the others in the group. The therapist will also need to ask simple questions and be willing to restate these questions several times.

Topic selection usually does not pose any problems since the array of topics is not encumbered by the diagnosis of Alzheimer's disease. Step one is presented in the typical fashion as with any other group. Step two may include (depending on the level of disability) more questions that the seasoned therapist would normally use.

Some therapists have employed ten to twenty-five questions in groups of Alzheimer's disease patients. On occasion a therapist can complete step one, ask twenty to twenty-five questions in step two and have clients read a poem, and complete step five with clients in the second stage of Alzheimer's.

Step three of remotivation requires the therapist to continue to utilize easy-to-answer questions to explore the topic. In step three the therapist should be very active since clients will be answering with one- or two-word responses, yes and no responses, and rambling responses that will need to be restated. The therapist will need to intervene frequently to make the client's responses meaningful and understandable thereby creating a successful experience for clients. Step four again must be kept simple; hands-on work should be provided, such as rolling cookie dough, folding napkins, rolling pennies, petting a dog, feeding fish, and raking leaves. The therapist needs to remember that performing these tasks is more important than the quality of the work or the end product. The clients should always be encouraged to read during a session, especially the poem. The ability of an Alzheimer's patient is maintained well into the later stages of the disease. The client might not understand what he or she is reading but nevertheless will be able to read and therefore be able to contribute to the group.

SUMMARY

Remotivation therapy can successfully be utilized with Alzheimer's clients. It will not cure the disease but it will aid in reducing or preventing excess disability due to disuse. It will work optimally when the patients are receiving appropriate medications for their cognitive problems and behavioral problems. It requires involvement by the therapist. The therapist who expands the effort to utilize remotivation therapy will readily see outcomes that reward the client and the therapist.

A sample session is presented here to give the reader a sense of how remotivation can be utilized with an Alzheimer's patient. Many variations on the same session are possible.

Remotivation Therapy Sample Session

Sample Sessions Key: Client having a problem answering = (chpa)
Therapist = (thr)

Step One: Climate of acceptance
Step Two:
What is your favorite flower? (Chpa: Give choice) A rose or a daisy?
What is your favorite day of the week? (Chpa) (Thr) Name the day.
What animals are on a farm? (Chpa) (Thr) Name some animals. (Give plenty of verbal reward for every attempt made by client.)
Did you have a pet?
What was the pet's name?
(Therapist can respond and tell a story about his or her pet.)
What animal is man's best friend? (Chpa) (Thr) Give clue—is it a dog?
(If client wants to discuss responses, allow it.)
State that we are talking about dogs.
Who would like to read this poem with me?
Step Three:
Where does a dog sleep at night?
What does a dog eat?
What are some breeds or types, such as a bulldog?
(Show pictures of dogs.) Did you have a dog like this?
What noises does a dog make? (Thr) Demonstrate.
Who took care of your dog?
Step Four:
Is it hard work taking care of a dog?
Have you ever fed a dog?
Did you feed him or her from the table?
Did you ever brush a dog?
Was it hard?
Did you like it?
(Bring in a dog and let everyone who wants to brush the dog.)
Was that fun?
Step Five: Climate of appreciation

Comments on Sample Session

- Step one could have been continued to include more questions leading to the topic of dogs.
- After the reading, a step five could be completed.
- The therapist is active giving clues, responding to his or her own questions, filling in blanks, or prompting the client(s).

REFERENCES

American Psychiatric Association (2000). *Diagnostic and Statistical Manual of Mental Disorders,* Fourth Edition, Text Revision. Washington, DC: American Psychiatric Association.

Handy, C., Ronald, T., James, C., Warren, M., and Lancaster, M. (1994). *Alzheimer's Disease: A Handbook for Caregivers,* Second Edition. St. Louis, MO: Mosby-Year Book, Inc.

Hellen, C.R. (1998). *Alzheimer's Disease Activity-Focused Care.* Boston, MA: Andover Medical Publications.

Medina, J. (2000). *What You Need to Know About Alzheimer's.* Irving, CA: Psychiatric Times, Inc.

Sabat, R.S., and Collins, M. (1999). Intact social, cognitive abilities, and selfhood: A case study of Alzheimer's disease. *American Journal of Alzheimer's Disease,* 14(1), 11-19.

Chapter 14

Beneficial Blending of Remotivation Therapy and Recreation/Activity Therapy

Nancy Farmer

INTRODUCTION

Over the years, the faces and abilities of nursing home residents have changed. There was a time when people went into a nursing home when their families could no longer provide the assistance they required. This meant that assistance was needed only for ADLs (activities of daily living—bathing, dressing, grooming). There were other facilities for people with mental/emotional impairments.

Today, with the closing of many state mental hospitals and the advent of home health care programs and assisted living facilities, clients are coming to long-term care facilities with myriad infirmities and abilities, both physical and psychological. In most cases, these infirmities have reached end-stage status before residents/clients enter one of these programs.

Activity professionals are faced with the task of providing for the psychosocial well-being of residents placed in our care. This is not an easy challenge. Three steps must be taken before decisions are made, which affect the way an individual's needs are met. These steps are

1. establish a rapport,
2. obtain a complete and accurate health and physical assessment, and
3. participate in the development of a plan of care.

One scenario that is experienced by health care providers includes the following:

1. Assess past history, both clinical and personal.
2. Assess client's abilities and limitations. Work with abilities not disabilities.
3. Interview client and/or family members about past interests.
4. Decide on a plan of care using information provided in steps one to three.

Accurate assessments are often made more difficult by the emotional status of the incoming residents. They are usually angry over losses suffered prior to admission—spouse/caregiver, home, physical/mental abilities, job, or purpose. When asked, most would reply "job or purpose" as being the worst loss of all.

Instead of living in a large house or apartment with family, they are now relegated to half a room and a stranger to share that room. They are told when to get up, eat, bathe, go to bed, and even when to use the bathroom! On the day of arrival, they are subjected to a complete "body check" and asked many personal questions. For independent, devout, private people, this is yet another great loss to their dignity.

USES OF REMOTIVATION THERAPY

Remotivation therapy can be used effectively, in group or individual sessions, to help facilitate the transition to nursing home placement. The following is an example of how remotivation therapy might be implemented to ease individuals' transition to their new environment/living situation:

1. *Climate of acceptance:* Introduce to staff and other residents, offer emphasis on past accomplishments, give positive affirmations. Provide reality orientation—use facility name often during tour/introductions. Bring them to their new circle of friends. Introduce to persons with similar backgrounds, interests, and abilities. (Know your group.) Coffee hour is usually their first success (and it also stimulates the thalamus).
2. *Poetry/song:* Use of appropriate background music for activity (hymns for spiritual activities, Mitch Miller for reminiscence, dance music, etc.).

3. *Provide objective subjects/activities of interest in a "no-fail" environment:* Allow residents the opportunity to participate or observe. Make sure to include them in the activity, if only as an observer.
4. *Eventually provide subjective activities:* Encourage success through past experience. Continue even if adaptive equipment is required. Allow time to achieve success and for clients to share their "work of the world."
5. *Climate of appreciation:* Invite to future activities and ask about other activities they would like to do/have. Always thank them for their participation and input.

One must always take into consideration that our clients/residents were all productive members of society. They all had formal education or on-the-job training. They are a wealth of knowledge and, when given the opportunity, are willing to share that knowledge. We must take care not to infantalize them by calling them honey, deary, sweetie, etc., or take over tasks they are capable of doing. Even though it may take them longer to accomplish these tasks, they should be given the opportunity to achieve success.

Residents need to be empowered by being provided with choices whenever possible. Federal guidelines regulate medication times, mealtimes, etc., but by offering choices, some level of control is afforded the client.

Activities/recreation therapy is the perfect venue for offering choice and empowerment. Some components of an activity program, which provides a better quality of life for the residents, are the following:

- *Empowerment:* Receipt/sending of mail, singing, newsletter committee, resident council, community outings, shopping trips/service, resident talent shows, craft fairs, raffle sales, skits and plays, and remotivation therapy
- *Spiritual:* Mass, worship service, Bible study, rosary, temple, hymn sings, Bible study tapes, Bible on tape, pastoral visits, and remotivation therapy
- *Intellectual:* bookmobile, museum trips, slide presentations, outside speakers, computer/art/other classes, and remotivation therapy

- *Educational:* art classes, computer classes, diversity training, GED for seniors, photography classes, and remotivation therapy
- *Creative:* crafts, woodworking, photography, gardening, watercolor classes, bell choir, sculpting, rhythm band, music, singing, and remotivation therapy
- *Social:* parties, musicals, coffee hour, patio parties, pool parties, theme parties/meals, and remotivation therapy

It is worth noting that remotivation therapy encompasses the whole spectrum of recommended components for effective activity programs. That is what makes it an invaluable tool for activity/recreation therapists.

A remotivation therapy session has all the elements required for an effective activity program. The group setting provides for sociability and, subsequently, the making of friends and bonding with friends and staff. The subjects provoke thoughts and provide intellectual and educational stimulation for participants. Group participation ensures empowerment and choice. The physical aspects of a remotivation group include walking/wheeling to group, handshaking, and the realization of five senses—auditory, tactile, gustatory, olfactory, and visual. The spiritual piece falls into play when participants reach into self and share experiences and ideals with others. Creativity is experienced through the use of poetry, songs, and making small crafts/pictures, etc.

REMOTIVATION AND MOVING EXPERIENCE

The structured remotivation therapy group is most effective, but variations can be presented for lower functioning residents. A "Moving Experience" program is designed specifically to stimulate the five senses—visual/sight, tactile/touch, auditory/hearing, gustatory/taste, olfactory/smell. This group is set up as any remotivation therapy group—a circle with the facilitator in the center—providing social contact for extremely low-functioning clients, who would ordinarily be confined to their rooms.

Appropriate music or sound effects playing in the background sets the stage for the topic/program of the day. This provides the auditory portion of the therapy and enhances the residents' quality of life. Appropriate snacks relating to the subject are made available, such as berries, juice, cotton candy, yogurt, and ice cream, which stimulate the thalamus and contribute the gustatory portion of the process. In addition to food, pine/balsam bags, colognes, potpourri, and flowers relate to the subject matter and provide for the olfactory portion of the therapy.

Tactile stimulation is provided through the use of hand creams/ hand massage, stuffed/or real animals, flowers, shells, etc. Items are passed from participant to participant/hand to hand. Touch can be healing in and of itself.

Visual aids are provided, which are appropriate to the subject. Eye contact is achieved staff to client and client to client. This promotes socialization, recognition of staff and peers and items, and provides mental stimulation to those participating in the group.

Process

The facilitator moves from client to client, speaking in a soft, nonthreatening manner, providing sensory stimulation as outlined previously. Reality orientation is also provided during these sessions—month, day, year, place, weather, and season. Topics are always seasonally appropriate.

Case studies have shown that participants who are involved in these one-hour sessions have shown an increase in awareness, improved facial affect, and an increase in abilities over time. They have shown a decrease in disruptive/negative behaviors and they have an increased tolerance for hands-on care. A few "case study" residents have resumed one-word responses after long periods of regression and silence.

The use of remotivation therapy with Alzheimer's and other dementia-related disorders requires shorter, more frequent sessions (daily if possible). Their attention spans have diminished, they tend to be disruptive in groups, and they are more apt to wander off during groups.

The use of music and songs, instead of poetry, works best with these residents/clients. Seasons, flowers (roses in particular), dolls, toys, cooking, home, and patriotic sessions are very successful topics relative to regressing mental abilities.

Residents should be placed at a round table with the facilitator (this discourages wandering). Give each person a hands-on project relating to the subject (snap peas/beans, peel carrots, take leaves off flowers, arrange flowers in vase, set table, grind coffee, turn handle on ice cream freezer, and similar projects). The sorting of buttons, stamps, socks, and coins, etc., works well in the first stages of the disease process. Stacking items, holding animals, folding laundry, and winding yarn are also very successful interventions for these residents.

Structure is also very important and the same pattern should be followed daily. The clients will follow your lead and, in time, know what is expected. They feel secure with rote activities. Play hymns at the beginning. They will sit down, as if in church. Play our national anthem at the end and they will all stand. They are a very devout and patriotic generation.

ACTIVITIES BLENDED
WITH REMOTIVATION THERAPY

Reminiscence is a natural blend for remotivation. Visual aids, pictures, music, conversations, reliving past experiences, and emotions are involved. These are all components of both reminiscence and remotivation therapy. Residents are asked to share their life experiences, memories, and personal possessions. When this happens, self-esteem is inevitably raised.

Ladies' teas are a perfect venue for remotivation. The table is set, tea and cookies served (stimulating the thalamus), introductions made (climate of acceptance established), and reality orientation provided. Bounce questions are asked and the subject established. Poetry is read pertaining to the subject, helping the clients use an undamaged portion of the brain. Steps three and four are accomplished with pertinent visual aids. The tea ends with thanks, handshakes, and the establishment of future topics solicited from the participants (climate of appreciation accomplished). Clients leave the group looking forward to their next tea, for which a specific date and time is decided upon. This is another opportunity for empowerment and choice.

Men's group is preferably led by a male; masculine topics/activities are pursued. Men miss their jobs and being "in charge" so, in an environment where female domination prevails, keeping them feeling good about themselves is not an easy task. It stands to reason that pizza parties, sports nights, poker night, fishing, woodworking, and antique cars are very successful. Utilizing the remotivation therapy format enhances camaraderie and promotes social interaction and self-esteem among the participants.

The versatility of remotivation therapy is endless. One-on-one remotivation is very successful for the self-isolating resident. The technique is nonthreatening and patient specific, a term used often when establishing good care plan goals. The family members must be included in this process. They can provide valuable information about the client/resident, which will help the facilitator establish the subject matter for future sessions, ensuring that the topics will be well received. Once a trusting relationship is built, most residents will venture out and begin interacting with others on their own.

Boredom, sensory deprivation, and depression are known to contribute to premature death in the elderly. Remotivation therapy can reduce this statistic.

Chapter 15

Variables to Consider When Establishing a Remotivation Group with the Domiciliary Care Population

Cheryl Davis

Even with the most homogeneous mixture of participants, many variables need to be considered when establishing any new therapy group. However, imagine the possibility of variables in establishing a remotivation group in a care facility when you consider the rapidly changing demographics of the domiciliary care environment. The range of residents could encompass seniors with dementia, middle-aged individuals with developmental disabilities, fairly young men and women dually diagnosed with mental illness and substance abuse, individuals cognitively intact with physical disabilities, or any combination of the former. How does one organize such a group? Whom does one include, and whom does one exclude? This is especially complex when the treatment modality has been documented as an effective application for each distinct group.

Here are some suggestions as to what you should consider when planning your remotivation therapy group. There are no definitive right or wrong approaches, although some have been proven more successful than not in the majority of cases. However, by outlining the possible variables for consideration as well as the pros and cons of each, it is hoped that group leaders working with rest home or nursing home inhabitants can develop a "personalized" group, appropriate for their clientele and situation. This can be done by identifying the strengths, needs, and interests of both the remotivator and group members, as well as by realistically accessing the resources available to them in their respective communities.

THE CLASSIC REMOTIVATION GROUP

This is the type of remotivation typically associated with nursing home and other institutionalized patients as originally conceived by Dorothy Hoskins Smith and practiced by Walter Pullinger Jr. The purpose of the therapy and the expected outcome is that the patient will be less withdrawn and isolated. It is also expected that the recipient of this therapy will be at least minimally more verbal, but preferably more responsive in general. Any remotivator can tell you that this is a very effective treatment tool. I have not met one who has not been amazed at how this seemingly simple approach has impacted even the most nonresponsive, severely institutionalized individual. Although it is difficult to improve on perfection, certain "trade" tricks are likely to add double insurance to the already fail-safe traditional remotivation format.

"I've Got the Time and the Place"

Probably the single most effective strategy to establishing a new group when trying to follow the classic remotivation structure is holding the group in the same common area of the facility and during the same time slot. Upon selection of the time and space, individuals you have identified as prospective group members should be notified of when the group will be held. Traditional target groups are ideal— long-term mental health patients who have exchanged addresses at state hospitals for private facility beds and withdrawn seniors suffering from dementia and/or depression.

Selection of the area in which the group is to be held is very important. If the group is in an area that is difficult to access or too remote, you will lose the individuals who will originally tell you they will not attend, but then meander on the sidelines to check out the group before committing to participation. Obviously, if the area is too busy and has too much traffic, the group will be distracted frequently. Still, in nursing homes and rest homes activities and groups are often held in large, common areas where several activities occur concurrently.

An example of such would be a dining area where the rattle of pots and pans being washed can be heard even when no meal is in progress. Aside from the inevitable diversions that will occur when using such an area, an additional disadvantage is the lack of natural barriers to limit the number of participants. As any remotivator can attest, once a group has been established, attendance often skyrockets. Remotivation provides a nonthreatening atmosphere in which individuals can express themselves without criticism and is preferable to the monotony of the rest home.

As a result, the numbers of those previously mentioned meanderers are likely to steadily increase. The ideal location within the facility will be a room or small waiting area that comfortably holds approximately ten people. The area need not have a door, but should be at least partially enclosed. It should be both easily and handicapped accessible.

Once the group begins to meet at the regularly scheduled day, time, and place, you will be able to measure its increasing success by the number of people who gather without prompting at the allotted place and day at the approximate time the group is expected to meet.

"Let Me Tell You 'Bout the Flowers and the Trees"

Establishing a routine meeting place and time will ensure that bona fide group members and interested but uncommitted residents know when and where to find you. Even dementia victims will place you on that internal time clock that science has yet to unravel—they will not know what today's date is, but they will come sit in the waiting area at the day and time you have identified twenty minutes before group is scheduled to begin. However, the key to keeping them coming will be the topics covered in your sessions and how completely you have achieved the climate of comfort and acceptance. Although a large degree of flexibility is allowed in the former, the latter cannot be compromised.

The most triumphant remotivator will intuitively choose topics that are geared to the interests and skill level of the group participants. In most cases, it will not even matter if all the group members have had any firsthand experience with the group's theme. If the topic has general applications to the lives of all, the questions asked are appropriate and not partial, and a true climate of acceptance has been previously instituted, almost any topic will be acceptable. However, the strongest topics for dementia and chronically mentally ill individuals will be those that stir strong memories or opinions, much in the way that reminiscent therapy does.

I recently attended a newly formed group as a guest. The topic was "pets." It was a very good topic for a traditional group with traditional participants. Most of the women were extremely enthusiastic about the session's theme, but one admitted that she had never owned a pet, and had very little interest in animals in general.

As the group progressed, she was increasingly outspoken about her conservative views about pets and how they should be maintained in the home. This is representative of how an appropriately chosen topic coupled with a firmly entrenched climate of acceptance will keep a group intact in what might normally be uncomfortable situations. Although this lady had no personal experience with pets, she did have a general knowledge of pets and enough familiarity to have formed opinions. Most important, the atmosphere of the group had been developed in such a way that she became aware as the discussion continued that she could express those minority opinions without reprisal.

Remarkably, I later learned that this was her first remotivation session. During this one experience, she became aware of and utilized the true advantages of this type of therapy. *Never* underestimate the importance of the climate of acceptance, particularly when trying to develop a new group. It is the key to remotivation, and the lack of it will nullify and eventually destroy an otherwise perfectly planned session. This is why it is important to follow the remotivation format as it is taught in the beginner's course without exception when doing a classic remotivation group.

Safeguards of the climate of acceptance are built into the remotivation process. Although it is comforting to all possible group participants, this fragile population is most dependent on it. Following the basic outline provides the most protection when doing the traditional remotivation session.

"It Don't Mean a Thing If It Ain't Got That Swing"

The poem has become known as the standard fare of the remotivation therapy session and is certainly an adaptable group aid. Several poems are available on every topic, varying from simplistic to symbolic; when you can't find one, you can make one up. The truly innovative remotivator will augment the traditional poem with a less traditional, more creative, visual/sensory aid. Virtually, the sky is the limit.

Only the remotivator's own imagination, time guidelines, and budget are restricting factors.

A group about ice cream can include questions about food preferences and sundae fixings and end with group members making a sundae to their own specifications. A group on smell can include group members trying to identify smells in paper bags. A group on pictures can provide group members with an opportunity to take a Polaroid picture. The possibilities are endless.

Remotivation can be used to add verbal fullness to already planned arts and crafts type activities provided in most care facilities. A group done on jewelry can end with group members making a jewelry box out of Popsicle sticks.

An added benefit to adding an arts and crafts component to a regularly scheduled remotivation group is that it usually engages staff as completely as it engages residents. Other staff members will soon meander to where group is being held to see what today's topic is and what the accompanying visual/sensory aid is as well. They will assist you if time permits and frequently start coming by at the regularly scheduled time to see if you need support. The experience will give them the opportunity to see patients they usually only see as regressed in a totally different light.

"Paying the Piper"

If you work for the facility and have no accountability to an outside accounting source, you can merrily skip over this section. Most remotivators, however, must report to Medicaid, Medicare, or some private insurance provider. Somewhere in the evolution of remotivation, therapists got the impression that remotivation is not a viable billing modality. Where this originated and why it persists is unclear. Decreased withdrawal as evidenced by increased verbalization and maintenance of basic life skills despite living in an institutional setting are valid treatment goals. They are, coincidentally, conventional remotivation goals. Remotivators need to clearly document the goals of the treatment as well as how progress toward the goal will be measured. This is standard documentation for every type of therapy and not specific to remotivation only. Remotivators who follow guidelines for proper documentation should not have any problems with reimbursement for services. Of course, remotivators must also meet the educational and accreditation requirements of the particular insurance they are trying to bill.

"FYI"

Occasionally you may be confronted with individuals who are so truly regressed that they are not ready for the group process. Although modern remotivators tend to think of the method only as a group process, remember that Dorothy Hoskins Smith began by reading poetry to patients in their beds and asking for their impressions of what she had just read. What worked then continues to work now; remotivation can still be used to reach out to the seemingly catatonic or extremely depressed individual. When the therapist thinks the patients have improved, they can then be moved on to the group process.

THE DOUBLE TROUBLE (DUAL DIAGNOSIS) GROUP

Once your weekly group has been established, you will notice that your group is attracting a set of participants who would not have even been considered appropriate for rest home placement twenty years ago. This resident is typically younger, mentally ill, more cognitively intact, physically able, and might actually be capable of living in the community if it were not for a substance abuse problem and resultant homelessness. These patients recently have been receiving a considerable amount of attention in the mental health professional community, as well as some nominal funding because of the difficulties that are unique in their treatment.

Although other therapies have had limited outcomes, one that has had greater success with this population has been remotivation. They like remotivation because they are not judged in the therapy process and because it provides an outlet in the usually boring routine associated with domiciliary living. This is particularly true because they are typically placed in rest homes and family care homes that are in a rural location, the rationale being that in most cases this limits their accessibility to the preferred substance of abuse. In addition, activities planned in the facility are usually geared toward the more typical rest home resident.

The mentally ill substance abuser (MISA) is ready for and responds very dramatically to the nurturing and educational aspects of remotivation. It can be used in myriad ways in clinical treatment and social reintegration.

Criticized as either "crazy" or "druggies," and undesirable in either case, these particular residents have had constant reminders of their inadequacies. Their failings have been made apparent to them in their dealings with the many systems on which they are dependent. The nurturing of the "wounded self" builds self-confidence and provides a backdrop in which the residents will feel comfortable facing issues they have been avoiding.

Once this phenomenon has occurred, you will literally know more than you want to know. Whether this is the group you had originally identified to provide remotivation or you have decided to start a second group that caters more to the needs of the MISA patients because of their interest in your initial group, you will find it a rewarding and versatile experience.

"Any Time, Any Place," or "Taking to the Streets"

The lack of activity at the facility, coupled with the cognitive abilities of these residents and their overall higher functioning, makes the MISA group perfect for the psychoeducational components of remotivation. Their physical capabilities free you from the confines of the home. Of course, you will need to decide how comfortable you are in exercising that freedom. How well you know members of your group, whether you have staff other than yourself to assist, time barriers, cost, transportation, and other resources should be examined when making your decision. Let's face it: the field trip is not for everybody. However, if you can pull this one off, even occasionally, it will be well worth your effort.

Although meeting at the same time and same place will strengthen the more traditional group, venturing outside the confines of the facility on occasion will energize the dual diagnosis group. That is not surprising when you consider that the average age of the MISA patient in a facility is early forties. How many people in the general population and same age range would be content to sit idle most of their day? The change of scenery can be just that, a change of scenery, while engaging in the group process. However, for the truly industrious it can serve as a visual/sensory aid to the identified topic.

If you decide that you would like to engage in activities outside of the facility as a visual/sensory aid to your topic, you may find that you need to be flexible with the time your group is held.

I personally think this is good experience for the remotivation patient who still has the cognitive ability to discern and adjust to time changes, and may be capable of leaving the semi-institutional life of the rest home, nursing home, or family care facility. Life outside the state hospital and the rest home does not run on an exact time schedule. Appointments at clinics, doctor's offices, the department of social services, and the Social Security Administration, for example, are likely to be scheduled on an availability basis.

The goal for many of these patients is stabilization and return to the least restrictive environment with supportive services. In the community environment, they will not find a noncompromising daily routine, and will need to be flexible.

"Let Me Tell You 'Bout the Birds and the Bees"

Your most pressing dilemma will most likely be that you, the remotivator, will need to decide what you would like to concentrate your efforts on, and what will be most relevant to your prospective participants. You can approach the development of your groups in many ways, and the sophistication of the MISA clients and their "been there, done that" attitudes can present a special challenge to the remotivator.

I suggest that you begin the sessions with these higher functioning residents with the same type of topics you utilize with your lower functioning groups. Let's say, for example, that you decide you still want to concentrate on the basic remotivation goals of encouraging less isolation and more verbalization. A group on bowling could take place at an actual bowling alley with group members either watching other people bowl or attempting to do so themselves as the visual/sensory aid. The original objectives of remotivation have been maintained but by providing an out-of-facility visual aid, either with physical activity or without, you have provided the MISA patient with a memory, a challenge, or the opportunity to try something new.

Now consider a new scenario with the same previously mentioned session on ice cream. Your session requires at least some minor revision. Instead of (or in addition to) questions about the group's favorite flavors and condiments, more thought-provoking questions should also be included.

Consider the following as an example: What health conditions would limit the amount of ice cream a person might eat? Name one vitamin or mineral that is found in ice cream. Name something about ice cream that has changed in the past ten years. As a visual/sensory aid the group could make homemade ice cream. This will be a hands-on demonstration of what ingredients to put into ice cream and the process that produces this treat. Do you want to show by example the changes within the ice cream industry? A trip to Baskin-Robbins or any local ice cream parlor will demonstrate that. What are the new flavors? What is in them? Follow up with a quick zip through the supermarket. How many bowls of ice cream from a half-gallon container could you eat for the same price as a Häagen-Dazs bar? This is how you begin to embrace the psychoeducational component to group.

The educational quality of remotivation therapy is apparent in this example. It can be used in single topic groups such as this one on ice cream or in a theme-related string of prepared topics.

Substance abuse is one area where the positive effects of remotivation are beginning to be recognized. As substance issues are going to be common to all the participants as either current, past, or at-risk users, a series of groups developed on this broad topic could be representative of this technique. For example, the first session might have "prescribed drug" as the chosen topic, and the second might have a "street drugs" topic. The third session might be on "relapse and relapse prevention." The fourth session might be on "the effects of drug addiction on health."

Another group may focus on the effects of social interactions. A group that highlights how actively using drugs interferes with living independently may follow it. Still another may focus on how drug addiction plays a role in the transmission of AIDS and other sexually transmitted diseases. The possibilities of "bounce," "sharing the world," and "work appreciation" questions are endless. Once again, a limited imagination on the part of the remotivator will be the only barrier to the many opportunities.

When you begin to do remotivation with a higher functioning group and/or disseminate fundamental information through the psychoeducational format, you are beginning to move into the realm of advanced remotivation. When utilizing advanced techniques, the remotivator still must maintain the climate of acceptance. As the topics may more frequently uncover "wounded" areas, it remains imperative that questions be asked in the more general "What might a person do?" providing the patients the anonymity they might wish to maintain. Even using this ploy, you will find that the majority of your responses will be answered in the first person, but that will have been the participant's choice.

Also remember that the group itself and the visual aids chosen to accompany the group to be indicative of the topic are voluntary endeavors. You may encourage the patient to participate but in order to maintain the true climate of acceptance, the participation should be voluntary.

"More Bounce to the Ounce"

A prepared and creative remotivator can provide a variety of visual aids in lieu of or in conjunction with the customary poem. Let's look more closely at the substance abuse psychoeducational model that we developed in the last section and the visual/sensory aids that can be utilized to enhance the remotivation and learning process.

If the remotivator has a basic knowledge of the prescribed medical and psychiatric drug regimen adhered to by the group members, he or she can have handouts available on the purpose for taking the drug, the side effects that may accompany usage, and the risk (if any) of drug interactions. That second group on street drugs might include a video that demonstrates the social, economic, and physical effects of continued substance use. The third scheduled group on relapse and relapse prevention might include a visit to a local NA or AA group as the visual sensory aid. A guest speaker from the health department can do a presentation of the effects of drug usage on major organs and body systems to provide supporting information on the physical effects of abuse. The results of these former two groups would be not only the psychosocial benefit, but also the expansion of the participant's community awareness and support system.

You can think of other therapeutic options (such as role-playing) and community resources (such as police, parole, and churches) that can be pulled in to assist in the psychoeducational remotivation process. Adding this level of visual/sensory aid to the group process requires advance planning, but the results are impressive and long lasting, as the participants will remember more of what has been introduced at the session.

Another advantage to a theme-developed psychosocial treatise of issues is its repetitive (although not obviously so) nature. With the group topics being somewhat intertwined, some of the same major concepts are likely to surface intermittently. This is beneficial because much learning can take place through repetition.

THE STAFF DEVELOPMENT GROUP

Remotivation is an excellent method to use for training facility staff as the psychoeducational and nurturing benefits that apply to the residents apply equally to the staff. The sessions are designed in the same manner as any other session with jump questions leading to the topic, followed by a visual/sensory aid and questions intended to describe and provide illumination of the topic. Another visual/sensory aid may be included or the group may simply end with questions that provide insight on how the topic applies to the workings of the "real" world.

EPILOGUE

Recently a colleague and I were invited to provide training at a local nursing home on how staff can use attitude as a behavior management tool. It was an extremely large group, and we had not been prepared for that; but we decided to follow the remotivation format as we had planned.

There were easily sixty in attendance, and at least half of them had no apparent interest in being there. Expecting a lecture, you can imagine their surprise when we began by saying hello to each of them individually, gave them the customary compliment, and then proceeded to ask them questions. By the time we had reached the poem, the group had relaxed considerably. Only one person in the room still appeared resistant to being there. Even she participated and responded to questions.

The others responded enthusiastically. There was laughter at some answers, bonding between the participants, and even a good-natured competition as individuals tried to come up with original answers. There was even subtle acknowledgment between participants when someone did manage a response that had not been uttered earlier when we went around the circle.

Due to the unexpected size of the group, we were in the "sharing the world" phase when it was brought to our attention that we had utilized almost all our time. We skipped to "the world of work" to ask a question about how all of this related to their work. They demonstrated that as a group they had an excellent understanding of what we were trying to relate, and presented some touching, worthwhile insights of their own.

Many stopped in groups on the way out to tell us how they had really enjoyed the training. They talked about how past trainings have usually been boring and asked if we performed any other types of training as they wanted to be included if possible.

This example is a testimony as to how remotivation can be used to provide information in a friendly environment, how it alters staff attitudes, and how it fosters relationships not only between participants, but also between the remotivator and the group members. Approximately three months after having done this one session in this nursing home in which I previously had no other dealings, I returned to see if they would lend their facilities for a remotivation training session. Although my hair had changed radically, and I had not seen any of them since, all of the staff who passed while I was making arrangements for the facility stopped to speak with me. One CNA introduced me to the nursing home director as "the only trainer who hadn't bored her to death" and instructed the director to get me back.

In the workplace, we sometimes feel like our patients frequently feel—as if we have no voice or any input into the policies and power structure that influence us daily. It is always rewarding when people seek our knowledge, opinions, and life experiences.

Chapter 16

The Role of Remotivation Therapy in Substance Abuse Prevention, Treatment, and Relapse Prevention

John R. Bierma

Substance abuse continues to be a major private and public health problem in all areas of the world. In 1992, the National Institute on Drug Abuse and the National Institute on Alcohol Abuse and Alcoholism of the National Institutes of Health estimated the cost of alcoholism and drug abuse to society at $246 billion, the most recent year for which sufficient data are available (Holland and Mushinski, 1999). With such high costs to society, a high priority of government has been to research methods of primary prevention, treatment, and relapse prevention.

During the early 1990s, the United States funded a series of major national comprehensive studies of substance abuse treatment called the national Drug Abuse Treatment Outcome Studies (DATOS) (Etheridge et al., 1999; Battjes, Onken, and Delany, 1999). The researchers looked at all aspects of the process of treatment, beginning with pretreatment variables, treatment models, and posttreatment relapse interventions.

PRETREATMENT VARIABLES

One of the studies cited previously looked at the factors prior to treatment that influence beginning treatment and long-term treatment success. The focus was on problem recognition, treatment readiness, sociodemographic indicators, drug use history and dependence, criminality, comorbid psychiatric diagnosis, and previous treatment.

Retention and engagement based on ratings of client and counselor relationships served as outcome criteria (Joe, Simpson, and Broome,

1998). The findings were somewhat surprising and revealing. Pre-treatment motivation was related to retention in all three modalities: long-term residential, outpatient methadone, and outpatient drug-free residential. The treatment readiness scale was the strongest predictor of long-term treatment and outpatient methadone treatment. Higher treatment readiness was significantly related to early therapeutic engagement in each modality.

The authors conclude that indicators of intrinsic motivation, especially readiness for treatment, were not only significant predictors of engagement and retention, but were more important than sociodemographic, drug use, and other background variables.

Another of these studies found that patients expressing greater confidence and commitment after three months of treatment generally began with higher motivation at intake, had formed better rapport with counselors, and attended counseling sessions more frequently (Broome, Simpson, and Joe, 1999).

Motivation for change plays a very important role in substance abuse treatment; it influences people to seek, complete, and comply with treatment, and make successful long-term changes in their behavior. As a result, researchers must take more seriously the role of motivation in the treatment of and recovery from substance abuse and to incorporate motivational enhancement strategies into treatment programs (DiClemente, Bellino, and Neavins, 1999).

The fundamental principle to create readiness for change and motivation for treatment is the presentation of "reality," or factual information, in an accepting, autonomy-supporting context. This process facilitates integration of the information into new behaviors that can be naturally maintained by the individual over time. If the context of information presentation is not supporting, but coercive or imposed socially from without, then the information is "internalized" in the form of guilt or social obligation. Research has shown that internalized behaviors are not naturally maintained by the individual over time and will be abandoned (Deci et al., 1994).

REMOTIVATION THERAPY

Remotivation therapy has been shown for over fifty years to be an effective individual and group motivational enhancement strategy (Pullinger, 1967; Holmes and Everline, 1984; Husaini et al., 1990;

Murphy, Conley, and Hernandez, 1994) that consists of five "steps." The steps of remotivation are described in nonjargon, metaphorical terminology to help the staff and clients of service agencies and hospitals better understand and apply the strategy in their personal interactions with clients (Bierma, 1998). The steps are

1. The Climate of Acceptance,
2. A Bridge to the Real World,
3. Sharing the World in Which We Live,
4. Appreciation of the Work of the World, and
5. The Climate of Appreciation.

The intent of this discussion is not to fully describe or inform the reader about the theoretical and research underpinnings of remotivation therapy. However, from the perspective of substance abuse treatment, certain qualities of remotivation therapy make it an ideal method to strategically incorporate into substance abuse prevention, treatment, and recovery.

Visual Representations

One of these qualities is part of the process in step two, A Bridge to the Real World. Step two employs a series of concrete, objective, and open-ended questions addressed to the client(s), which leads the focus of discussion to a predetermined topic or aspect of the real world. At this point in the session a verbal picture (poem) describing the topic is shared with the client(s). Pictures of the topic are also shared. If the topic is abstract in nature, the group leader will ask the client(s) to define the concept using words and metaphors from the poem or pictures or from their personal experiences with the concept.

Recent research in substance abuse treatment has shown that the use of diagrams or visual representation in the form of node-link pictures constructed by client(s) individually or as a group increases treatment outcomes (Dees, Dansereau, and Simpson, 1994; Pitre et al., 1998; Simpson et al., 1997; Newbern, Dansereau, and Pitre, 1999). Clients with less education have been shown to respond better to therapy that incorporates visual representations (mapping or node-linking) than to therapy that does not include it (Pitre, Dansereau, and Joe, 1996).

Acceptance

Another quality of remotivation therapy that is consistent with and supported by current research and theory in substance abuse is the concept of acceptance. The concept of acceptance is a fundamental principle of remotivation therapy that begins in step one, The Climate of Acceptance, and is maintained and enhanced throughout the remaining steps of a session. How acceptance is conveyed to the client(s) and how this step relates to associated concepts and behaviors should be understood.

Step one begins as the group or individual therapist looks at a client, making eye contact if possible, and says, " Hello, _____ (client's name), my name is _____ (therapist's name). I like _____(a non–personally embarrassing compliment is paid to the client, such as "I like the color of your blouse"). This simple introduction and statement accomplishes a couple of very important things. One, it recognizes the person as an individual with a name! This reinforces individual identity and autonomy. Second, paying an objective compliment communicates that your intent is not to be critical or judgmental. The questions that begin step two are impersonal and asked in terms of personal opinion so that all answers are "correct," such as what is your favorite color? The questioner always accepts the answer without judgment or editorial comment. The decision to answer belongs to the client and the answer is his or hers, accepted and respected by the therapist. This is modeled by the group therapist to other clients in a group session. This process of questioning and accepting is the primary process of remotivation therapy.

The behaviors just described are intensely supportive of client autonomy and they build intrinsic motivation (Ryan, Kuhl, and Deci, 1997; Deci et al., 1994).

Substance abuse treatment has had a long history of coercive methods. Many addicted people were put in drunk tanks "to sleep it off." Many states had laws that allowed civil commitment to a mental institution for the treatment of addiction. Many therapists and people in support recovery groups believed that addicts had to "hit bottom" psychologically and physically before they developed the motivation to seek treatment. This has led to interventions that are coercive and make the client hit bottom sooner than later! Current research shows that coercive methods do have positive outcomes but are not as effective as supportive, autonomy-producing methods (Miller, Meyers, and Tonigan, 1999). In light of this research, it is important to recognize that the degree of coerciveness perceived by clients is determined by the multiple social and psychological events leading to treatment. Some clients do not find mandatory treatment to be coercive, and some self-referred seemingly voluntary clients find their experience very coercive. If the legal system is autonomy supportive of the addict, he or she will find it noncoercive. Likewise, if a family has pressured a client psychologically, and isolated the client socially, he or she will find their voluntary admission to treatment as very coercive (Wild, Newton-Taylor, and Alletto, 1998).

Research in substance abuse treatment and in other disease treatments has found that the behaviors of individual therapists and programs that support client autonomy and autonomous behavior produce better and longer lasting outcomes in smoking cessation (Williams et al.,1999); weight loss (Williams et al.,1996); alcohol and drug treatment (Wild, Newton-Taylor, and Alletto, 1998); HIV infection risk behaviors (Carey et al., 2000); diabetes (Williams, Freedman, and Deci, 1998); schizophrenia (Aquila, Weiden, and Emanuel, 1999); and medication compliance (Williams et al., 1998).

Cost Effectiveness

Many of the programs and interventions that have been studied include highly paid professionals as direct service providers. This author's position is that great sums of public funds are wasted by paying highly educated persons to provide direct treatment. Motivation-enhancing strategies, such as remotivation therapy, need to be learned and used by professionals. They must possess the skills and understand remotivation in order to develop the most effective way to incorporate it into the overall treatment and recovery process.

Less educated professionals and laypeople such as family members, friends, case managers, caseworkers, nurse aides, and volunteers can learn motivation-enhancing strategies as effectively as professionals. Less formally educated persons may actually use the methods more effectively than professionals due to simple communication barriers such as vocabulary and cultural values that create a distance between therapist and client.

Implications

All of the previously mentioned research underscores some very important policy, programmatic, and therapeutic principles.

1. Short of science finding a genetic or one-time cure for addictions, if medications aid in the treatment of addictions, then the client must be motivated to take the medication.
2. If treatment continues to consist of behavioral interventions that require client voluntary participation, motivation will continue to be a prerequisite and determining factor in treatment outcome and ongoing recovery.
3. Funding sources will waste money on programs and medications if they do not pay for motivation-enhancing strategies as part of the overall process of care and ongoing support for relapse prevention.
4. Families and significant others, such as teachers, pastors, and employers, must learn the behavioral principles that support autonomy and intrinsic motivation so that primary prevention and relapse prevention can be cost effective.

Applications

Many health care providers have used remotivation therapy methods within the process of their care and treatment of persons with addictions. From personal experience, these health care providers came to training from all levels of education and came from many different disciplines. Some of the programs in which remotivation has been applied are summarized next.

Detoxification

Staff under the author's supervision at a hospital in Raleigh, North Carolina, conducted remotivation group sessions in the detoxification unit of a local substance abuse hospital. Length of stay was approximately two to four days. Clients experienced varying degrees of cognitive impairment and lack of concentration or attention. The group sessions provided an accepting, autonomy-supporting experience, which motivated the clients toward participation in self-help groups or treatment groups upon discharge.

Court-Ordered Drug Education Classes

DUI offenders who were receiving drug education classes under court order in North Carolina substance abuse treatment centers were presented information using remotivation as the delivery method for the information. In both centers, the clients rated the remotivation sessions more highly than lecture/discussion methods or psychodynamic problem-solving methods. Attendance during the eight mandatory sessions increased dramatically when remotivation methods were used and clients refrained from smoking during sessions. Remotivation produced better group outcomes by all standard measures used to internally evaluate staff and client response to sessions.

Substance Abuse Treatment

Staff at the treatment center in Rocky Mount, North Carolina, incorporated remotivation methods into their treatment program by inviting clients to attend eight weeks of remotivation sessions, followed by eight weeks of standard confrontive substance abuse group treatment, followed by eight weeks of psychoeducation on relapse prevention using a remotivation format.

Adolescent and Family Substance Abuse Treatment

The treatment center in Rocky Mount also used remotivation in its evening adolescent and family treatment program. The evening began with separate standard substance abuse treatment sessions for teens and for parents. Following a break, the parents and teens formed one group that was led using remotivation methods that focused on everyday topics to facilitate parent and teen communication and acceptance. These sessions were highly rated by both parents and teens for facilitating and modeling effective communication.

Substance Abuse Treatment Within the Remotivation Format of Group Work

In Greenville, New Bern, and Wilmington, North Carolina, substance abuse counselors were taught both "basic" and "advanced" remotivation methods. Therapists used remotivation as an alternative method of group process for their treatment sessions with clients. In many of the treatment sessions, the topics of the sessions to be covered in therapy were mandated by treatment guidelines, so the content of the sessions was identical to more traditional psychodynamic methods of treatment.

Therapists reported that clients rated the remotivation sessions more highly than traditional sessions. Attendance at group sessions increased dramatically and dropout rates declined. Research has shown that continued participation in treatment, regardless of the methods employed, is one of the largest predictors of abstinence. Therefore, group methods that increase attendance and reduce dropout rates from treatment are preferred.

REFERENCES

Aquila, R., Weiden, P.J., and Emanuel, M. (1999). Compliance and the rehabilitative alliance. *Journal of Clinical Psychiatry,* 60(19), 23-27.

Battjes, R.J., Onken, L.S., and Delany, P.J. (1999). Drug abuse treatment entry and engagement: Report of a meeting on treatment readiness. *Journal of Clinical Psychology,* 55(5), 643-657.

Bierma, J.R. (1998). *Remotivation Group Therapy: Handbook for the Basic Course.* York Harbor, ME: National Remotivation Therapy Organization, Inc.

Broome, K.M., Simpson, D.D., and Joe, G.W. (1999). Patient and program attributes related to treatment process indicators in DATOS. *Drug Alcohol Dependency,* 57(2), 127-135.

Carey, M.P., Braten, L.S., Maisto, S.A., Gleason, J.R., Forsyth, A.D., Durant, L.E., and Jaworski, B.C. (2000). Using information, motivational enhancement, and skills training to reduce the risk of HIV infection for low income urban women: A second randomized clinical trial. *Health Psychology,* 19(1), 3-11.

Deci, E.L., Eghrari, H., Patrick, B.C., and Leone, D.R. (1994). Facilitating internalization: The self-determination theory perspective. *Journal of Personality,* 62(1), 119-142.

Dees, S.M., Dansereau, D.F., and Simpson, D.D. (1994). A visual representation system for drug abuse counselors. *Journal of Substance Abuse Treatment,* 11(6), 517-523.

DiClemente, C.C., Bellino, L.E., and Neavins, T.M. (1999). Motivation for change and alcoholism treatment. *Alcohol Research & Health,* 23(2), 86-92.

Etheridge, R.M., Craddock, S.G., Hubbard, R.L., and Rounds-Bryant, J.L. (1999). The relationship of counseling and self-help participation to patient outcomes in DATOS. *Drug Alcohol Dependency,* 57(2), 99-112.

Holland, P. and Mushinski, M. (1999). Cost of alcohol and drug abuse in the United States, Alcohol/Drugs COI Study Team. *Statistical Bulletin, Metropolitan Insurance Companies,* 80(4), 2-9.

Holmes, E.A. and Everline, D. (1984). The use of volunteers in social group work as remotivation leaders. *Journal of Long Term Care Administration,* 12(4), 9-12.

Husaini, B.A., Castor, R.S., Whitten-Stovall, R., Moore. S.T., Neser, W., Linn, J.G., and Griffin, D. (1990). An evaluation of a therapeutic health program for the black elderly. *Journal of Health and Social Policy,* 2(2), 67-85.

Joe, G.W., Simpson, D.D., and Broome, K.M. (1998). Effects of readiness for drug abuse treatment on client retention and assessment of process. *Addiction,* 93(8), 1177-1190.

Miller, W.R., Meyers, R.J., and Tonigan, J.S. (1999). Engaging the unmotivated in treatment for alcohol problems: A comparison of three strategies for intervention through family members. *Journal of Consulting and Clinical Psychology,* 67(5), 688-697.

Murphy, M.C., Conley, J., and Hernandez, M.A. (1994). Group remotivation therapy for the 90s. *Perspectives in Psychiatric Care,* 30(3), 9-12.

Newbern, D., Dansereau, D.F., and Pitre, U. (1999). Positive effects on life skills motivation and self-efficacy: Node-link maps in a modified therapeutic community. *American Journal of Drug and Alcohol Abuse,* 25(3), 407-423.

Pitre, U., Dansereau, D.F., and Joe, G.W. (1996). Client education levels and the effectiveness of node-link maps. *Journal of Addictive Disturbances,* 15(3), 27-44.

Pitre, U., Dansereau, D.F., Newbern, D., and Simpson, D.D. (1998). Residential drug abuse treatment for probationers: Use of node-link mapping to enhance participation and progress. *Journal of Substance Abuse Treatment,* 15(6), 535-543.

Pullinger, W.F. Jr. (1967). A history of remotivation. *Hospital Community Psychiatry,* 18(1), 26-27.

Ryan, R.M., Kuhl, J., and Deci, E.L. (1997). Nature and autonomy: An organizational view of social and neurobiological aspects of self-regulation in behavior and development. *Developmental Psychopathology,* 9(4), 701-728.

Simpson, D.D., Joe, G.W., Rowan-Szal, G.A., and Greener, J.M. (1997). Drug abuse treatment process components that improve retention. *Journal of Substance Abuse Treatment,* 14(6), 565-572.

Wild, T.C., Newton-Taylor, B., and Alletto, R. (1998). Perceived coercion among clients entering substance abuse treatment: Structural and psychological determinants. *Addictive Behavior,* 23(1), 81-95.

Williams, G.C., Cox, E.M., Kouides, R., and Deci, E.L. (1999). Presenting the facts about smoking to adolescents: Effects of an autonomy-support style. *Archives of Pediatric Adolescent Medicine,* 153(9), 959-964.

Williams, G.C., Freedman, Z.R., and Deci, E.L. (1998). Supportive autonomy to motivate patients with diabetes for glucose control. *Diabetes Care,* 21(10), 1644-1651.

Williams, G.C., Grow, V.M., Freedman, Z.R., Ryan, R.M., and Deci, E.L. (1996). Motivational predictors of weight loss and weight maintenance. *Journal of Perspectives on Social Psychology,* 70(1), 115-126.

Williams, G.C., Rodin, G.C., Rayan, R.M., Grolnick, W.S., and Deci, E.L. (1998). Autonomous regulation and long-term medication adherence in adult outpatients. *Health Psychology,* 17(3), 269-276.

Chapter 17

Collaborative Team Models and Remotivation Therapy

Jean A. Dyer

INTRODUCTION

The interdisciplinary or multidisciplinary delivery of remotivation therapy requires collaboration among diverse health care disciplines. Collaboration in the delivery of health care has consistently remained the goal of direct care providers. Even though true collaborative delivery of therapeutic regimes remains a primary goal of many health care organization administrators, most find it very difficult to achieve this goal. Sullivan (1998) defined collaboration as a dynamic transforming process of creating a power-sharing partnership in health care practice, education, research, and organizational settings for the purposeful attending to client needs and problems in order to achieve likely successful outcomes. Sullivan also stated (1998, p. xiii),

> Collaboration requires of its practitioners the acquisition and application of a complex constellation of values and abilities. When two or more collaborators agree upon plans and actions a mutually satisfying and productive collaborative relationship may result. Such relationships, while not rare, are neither readily achieved nor maintained.

As early as 1965, Garber credited the success of remotivation therapy to the attributes of the clinical remotivators from varying health care disciplines. Garber recognized the discipline diversity from which remotivation therapy grew. He promoted the belief that remotivation therapy was successful because of the abilities, artful application, and presentation of the therapist, regardless of his or her title or condition of service (Garber, 1965).

Dorothy Hoskins Smith created the process of remotivation therapy in the late 1940s. With a background in English literature, Smith volunteered at a VA psychiatric hospital reading poetry to veterans. As a patient care attendant, Walt Pullinger Jr. continued to develop remotivation techniques following Smith's death. Pullinger authored the original poetry and twelve-week training program (Bierma, 1998).

Physicians and nurses became advocates for remotivation therapy under the auspices of the American Psychiatric Association in 1965 (Bierma, 1998). As practicing remotivation therapists, these physicians and nurses played an integral role in establishing remotivation therapy as a viable therapeutic regime in a variety of clinical settings.

Today, remotivation therapy is practiced by volunteers, certified nursing assistants, recreation and activity therapists, nurses, physicians, social workers, occupational therapists, counselors, chaplains, admissions staff, and health care administrators (Dyer, 2002). The application of remotivation therapy has also expanded beyond mental health hospitals. Remotivation therapy is effective in any health care setting where psychotherapy, rehabilitation, and patient education are primary components of the treatment plan. Such settings include substance abuse and behavioral health treatment facilities; assisted living, skilled nursing, and long-term care facilities; home care; adult day care; prisons; and jails (Dyer, 2002).

DEFINITIONS

The terms multidisciplinary and interdisciplinary are often used interchangeably, but inaccurately. The specifics of each of these concepts are important if health care delivery teams are to work effectively together. *Multidisciplinary* teams combine the skills and abilities of various discipline-specific health care providers. Hoeman (1996) stated, "Each discipline within a multidisciplinary team submits findings and recommendations, sets their own discipline-specific goals, and works within the discipline boundaries to achieve these goals independently" (p. 28).

Multidisciplinary teams maintain a sense of independence and uniqueness for each member of a discipline. However, conflict, competition, and turf issues create a team dynamic that can encourage duplication of effort, inconsistency in clinical outcomes, and poor client/team relationships (Hoeman, 1996). This very often produces uncooperative group dynamics that can drive up the cost of health care.

Health care providers meeting together to talk about a patient every week does not constitute a true team effort. Various team members may not fully participate or attend all the required meetings. Effective communication is extremely important because discipline-specific progress in the attainment of health care goals must be conveyed directly or indirectly to other team members (Hoeman, 1996). The success of the multidisciplinary health care plan is the product of the cumulative efforts of all the discipline-specific team members.

Interdisciplinary teams move beyond the parameters of each discipline. Each member of the team must be willing to respect the capabilities of other team members, trust them as colleagues, and work to create a common means of communication. The team must establish a common process for decision making that emphasizes the strengths of each discipline while minimizing the differences among those discipline-specific members of the team. Hoeman (1996) commented, "a team of professionals with different training, personalities, and particular expertise becomes cohesive with a common purpose and goal; the result is a smoothly functioning team that also happens to be a cost-effective team" (p. 79).

Interdisciplinary health care teams identify health care goals to be addressed by the team, rather than the health care plan being driven by multiple discipline-specific goals. This helps the team avoid duplication of effort or any conflict in goals. "Once the 'team goals' are identified, each discipline sets out to work toward goal attainment within the parameters of their discipline, collaborating when goals overlap discipline boundaries" (Hoeman, 1996, p. 28). Team members are involved in problem solving beyond the restrictions of their discipline (Diller, 1990).

Interdisciplinary health care teams are not only more effective in establishing a holistic clinical approach to client needs, they are more cost effective. Trust and confidence in one another is basic to establishing a commonality among professionals (Hoeman, 1996).

NATIONAL REMOTIVATION THERAPY
ORGANIZATION SURVEY RESULTS

In an effort to explore how remotivation therapy was being implemented in a variety of health care settings, a national survey sponsored by the National Remotivation Therapy Organization (NRTO) was completed by Dyer in August 2002.

One hundred and twenty-five active members of NRTO were surveyed. Forty-nine of the surveys (39 percent) were returned and analyzed. Seven practice settings were represented in the sample. These practice settings were long-term care, mental health, private practice, adult day care, assisted living, skilled nursing, and pastoral care. The multiple practice disciplines that were represented in the survey sample were consultants, activities, education, administration, nursing, psychology, pastoral care, counseling, occupational therapy, admissions, and social work.

Sixty-eight percent of the respondents were leading remotivation therapy groups at the time of the survey; 28 percent of those respondents led groups once a week or more. The majority of remotivation therapists surveyed were the only remotivation therapists in their facility. Most organizations employed one, two, or three health care providers who were certified in remotivation therapy. Only two organizations had eight or nine remotivation therapists in the same facility.

The survey was mailed to active members of the National Remotivation Therapy Organization. Demographic and informational data was collected for use in recruitment and retention efforts planned by NRTO. The following questions and results also provided preliminary basic information about the delivery of remotivation therapy in various health care settings.

> **Question:** Do you meet formally with other disciplines to discuss a patient's progress in remotivation sessions?
> **Responses:** Yes (35 percent), No (65 percent).
> **Question:** Where do you document your remotivation therapy process?
> **Responses:** Flow sheet (14 percent), nurses' notes (10 percent), physicians' notes (0 percent), other, e.g., progress notes, (53 percent), and 16 percent of the respondents did not document

their progress. Seven percent of those surveyed did not respond to this question.

Question: Do other team members implement remotivation therapy with the same patients as you do?

Responses: Yes (32 percent), No (51 percent), Did not respond (17 percent).

Question: If yes, do you cooperate in the delivery of remotivation therapy as a team?

Responses: Twenty-eight percent of the 32 percent responding "yes" indicated they cooperate with other disciplines. Ten percent of the respondents indicated they do not cooperate with other disciplines. Two percent did not indicate whether they cooperate.

Question: If you cooperate with other disciplines, what type of team approach do you use?

Responses: Of the total number of remotivation therapists surveyed, 33 percent used a cooperative approach to implement remotivation therapy.

Question: What are the primary barriers you believe inhibit the implementation of remotivation therapy in an interdisciplinary manner?

Responses: Not enough time, extensive paperwork, high patient/provider ratios, no financial reimbursement for health care facilities, the noticeable independence/competition among disciplines, resistance to change on the part of health care providers, and staffing shortages. The respondents also indicated a belief that remotivation therapy is not always taken seriously by administration, and that there was no universal identified need to train additional certified therapists in the facility.

DISCUSSION

Remotivation therapists continue to come from a diversity of health care disciplines. This supports the universality of remotivation therapy and its application to a variety of patients, clients, and residents in different health care settings.

Multidisciplinary and interdisciplinary health care teams are two cooperative delivery modalities used in various health care settings.

The data obtained from the survey support Sullivan's observation that acknowledged collaborative models, while not rare, are neither readily achieved nor maintained (Sullivan, 1998).

Presently, most health care providers deliver remotivation therapy through a multidisciplinary team. As indicated by Hoeman (1996), this cooperative approach allows each member of a given discipline to maintain his or her sense of independence, and affect discipline-specific health care outcomes. Survey data indicated that most remotivation therapists work independently or with one or two other remotivation therapists in their facility. Even when other team members were certified to implement remotivation therapy in the same facility, only 32 percent implemented remotivation therapy on the same patients/clients/residents.

In addition, only 28 percent of the therapists who implemented remotivation therapy indicated that they cooperate with other disciplines to deliver remotivation therapy as a team. Remotivation therapy appears to be considered a counseling technique that is dependent on the skill of the therapist rather then the cooperative skills of a health care team.

Communication is essential in multidisciplinary teams. According to the survey data, documentation of the remotivation therapy process appears to be inconsistent and at times nonexistent. Fourteen percent of the respondents document on flow sheets, 10 percent document in nurses' notes, and 53 percent designated the "other" category. None of the therapists documented patient/client/resident progress in the physicians' notes, and a surprising 16 percent did not document the remotivation process at all. These data suggest the need to formalize and standardize the implementation of remotivation therapy. Accurate and consistent documentation of this therapeutic regime is necessary to meet the accreditation and quality standards of care criteria established for health care delivery organizations.

The survey results suggested that health care providers are not required to consistently document the remotivation process in their facility or that therapists may not think what they do is important enough to document. This may be due to the identified perception that remotivation is not highly prioritized by many administrators in many health care organizations. In addition, remotivation is presently not reimbursed as an approved therapeutic regime and consequently is not required in the reporting process by accrediting or governmental organizations. Remotivation therapists strongly believe the process effectively supports the general well-being of a person, and they may be comfortable knowing their efforts serve the overall health care goal of achieving positive patient/client/resident health care outcomes.

To better provide the collaborative delivery of remotivation therapy in various health care settings, basic organizational dynamics must be addressed. The data obtained from this pilot study suggested a need for remotivation therapists to focus on development of remotivation therapy as a critical component of the health care plan.

To establish remotivation therapy as a generally accepted component of behavioral health care, remotivation therapists might consider

1. formulating a policy statement through the National Remotivation Therapy Organization that guides remotivation therapists in the course of insinuating themselves into a collaborative health care delivery process,
2. establishing an ongoing experiential educational process that would target administrators to increase their understanding of the cost-effective and behavioral health benefits associated with remotivation therapy,
3. creating a research-based resource for various disciplines to access when exploring behavioral health issues,
4. developing a speakers' bureau through the National Remotivation Therapy Organization to increase professional awareness regarding the benefits and versatility of remotivation therapy,
5. working through discipline-specific professional organizations to increase awareness on the part of health care professionals, and
6. establishing a lobby initiative at the state and federal levels that supports legislation to provide reimbursement for facilities that offer remotivation therapy to their patients/clients/residents.

These are bold steps requiring time and commitment on the part of each and every remotivation therapist presently involved in behavioral health. New remotivation therapists will need strong role models; health care organizations will need continued support through research and education. A strong national presence through the National Remotivation Therapy Organization will also need to be maintained. Are remotivation therapists up to the challenge of establishing remotivation therapy as an integral part of collaborative behavioral health care? The strong belief system and skills base evidenced by certified practicing remotivation therapists suggests this challenge can and will be met as the workplace becomes more collaborative.

REFERENCES

Bierma, J. (1998). *Remotivation Group Therapy: Handbook for the Basic Course.* York Harbor, ME: National Remotivation Therapy Organization, Inc.

Diller, L. (1990). Fostering the interdisciplinary team: Fostering research in a society in transition. *Archives of Physical Medicine and Rehabilitation, 71*, 275-278.

Dyer, J. (2002). National Remotivation Therapy Organization Survey, Paper presented at the meeting of the National Remotivation Therapy Organization Annual Institute, Ogunquit, ME, October.

Garber, R. (1965). A psychiatrist's view of remotivation. *Mental Hospitals,* August, 17-19.

Hoeman, S. (1996). *Rehabilitation Nursing: Process and Application.* St. Louis, MO: Mosby-Year Book, Inc.

Sullivan, T. (1998). *Collaboration: A Health Care Imperative.* New York: McGraw-Hill Companies, Inc.

Index

Page numbers followed by the letter "b" indicate boxed text.

Order a copy of this book with this form or online at:
http://www.haworthpress.com/store/product.asp?sku=5191

HANDBOOK OF REMOTIVATION THERAPY

_____in hardbound at $39.95 (ISBN: 0-7890-2470-5)

_____in softbound at $24.95 (ISBN: 0-7890-2471-3)

Or order online and use special offer code HEC25 in the shopping cart.

COST OF BOOKS_____

POSTAGE & HANDLING_____
*(US: $4.00 for first book & $1.50
for each additional book)*
*(Outside US: $5.00 for first book
& $2.00 for each additional book)*

SUBTOTAL_____

IN CANADA: ADD 7% GST_____

STATE TAX_____
*(NJ, NY, OH, MN, CA, IL, IN, & SD residents,
add appropriate local sales tax)*

FINAL TOTAL_____
*(If paying in Canadian funds,
convert using the current
exchange rate, UNESCO
coupons welcome)*

☐ **BILL ME LATER:** (Bill-me option is good on
US/Canada/Mexico orders only; not good to
jobbers, wholesalers, or subscription agencies.)

☐ Check here if billing address is different from
shipping address and attach purchase order and
billing address information.

Signature_____

☐ **PAYMENT ENCLOSED: $_____**

☐ **PLEASE CHARGE TO MY CREDIT CARD.**

☐ Visa ☐ MasterCard ☐ AmEx ☐ Discover
☐ Diner's Club ☐ Eurocard ☐ JCB

Account # _____

Exp. Date_____

Signature_____

Prices in US dollars and subject to change without notice.

NAME_____

INSTITUTION_____

ADDRESS_____

CITY_____

STATE/ZIP_____

COUNTRY_____ COUNTY (NY residents only)_____

TEL_____ FAX_____

E-MAIL_____

May we use your e-mail address for confirmations and other types of information? ☐ Yes ☐ No
We appreciate receiving your e-mail address and fax number. Haworth would like to e-mail or fax special
discount offers to you, as a preferred customer. **We will never share, rent, or exchange your e-mail address
or fax number.** We regard such actions as an invasion of your privacy.

Order From Your Local Bookstore or Directly From
The Haworth Press, Inc.
10 Alice Street, Binghamton, New York 13904-1580 • USA
TELEPHONE: 1-800-HAWORTH (1-800-429-6784) / Outside US/Canada: (607) 722-5857
FAX: 1-800-895-0582 / Outside US/Canada: (607) 771-0012
E-mailto: orders@haworthpress.com

For orders outside US and Canada, you may wish to order through your local
sales representative, distributor, or bookseller.
For information, see http://haworthpress.com/distributors

(Discounts are available for individual orders in US and Canada only, not booksellers/distributors.)
PLEASE PHOTOCOPY THIS FORM FOR YOUR PERSONAL USE.
http://www.HaworthPress.com   BOF04